LECTIN
AVOIDANCE
COOKBOOK

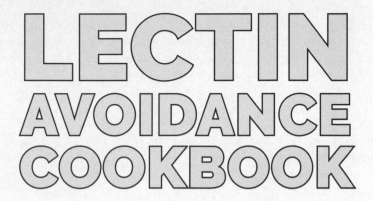

LECTIN AVOIDANCE COOKBOOK

150 Delicious Recipes to Reduce Inflammation, Lose Weight and Prevent Disease

Pamela Ellgen

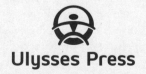

Ulysses Press

Published in the United States by:
ULYSSES PRESS
P.O. Box 3440
Berkeley, CA 94703
www.ulyssespress.com

ISBN: 978-1-61243-790-3
Library of Congress Control Number: 2018930781

Printed in Canada by Marquis Book Printing
10 9 8 7 6 5 4 3 2

Acquisitions editor: Bridget Thoreson
Managing editor: Claire Chun
Editor: Renee Rutledge
Proofreader: Shayna Keyles
Front cover design: David Hastings
Production: Jake Flaherty

Distributed by Publishers Group West

NOTE TO READERS: This book has been written and published strictly for informational and educational purposes only. It is not intended to serve as medical advice or to be any form of medical treatment. You should always consult your physician before altering or changing any aspect of your medical treatment and/or undertaking a diet regimen, including the guidelines as described in this book. Do not stop or change any prescription medications without the guidance and advice of your physician. Any use of the information in this book is made on the reader's good judgment after consulting with his or her physician and is the reader's sole responsibility. This book is not intended to diagnose or treat any medical condition and is not a substitute for a physician.

This book is independently authored and published and no sponsorship or endorsement of this book by, and no affiliation with, any trademarked brands or other products mentioned within is claimed or suggested. All trademarks that appear in ingredient lists and elsewhere in this book belong to their respective owners and are used here for informational purposes only. The author and publisher encourage readers to patronize the quality brands mentioned in this book.

CONTENTS

INTRODUCTION

A lectin-avoidance diet is nothing new. For thousands of years, humans have understood that certain compounds in foods are dangerous, and have figured out ways to avoid them. Soaking and sprouting grains and legumes, avoiding unripe fruits, tossing out green potatoes, peeling tough vegetables, avoiding certain plant seeds, and fermenting food to improve its digestibility are all ancient practices designed to maximize the benefits of healthy food and minimize the harmful effects. Global cultures have passed on these food traditions for millennia.

Modern Western food culture does not share this ethos. It is founded on what tastes good, what looks good, what has maximum profitability, and what will last the longest on the shelf. We don't really think about what our ancestors ate. Our food culture is transmitted through the television, not tradition.

Even more concerning, our diet is built around a handful of staple foods that are highly inflammatory and, in most cases, loaded with lectins—wheat, corn, soy, sugar, dairy, and meat. Oh, and our favorite vegetable: potatoes.

In toxicology, the underlying principle is that the dose makes the poison. Our doses of these foods are leaving us with unprecedented levels of overweight and obesity, metabolic syndrome, and autoimmune disorders.

Fortunately, there is a solution. And, as I hinted at before, it isn't all that groundbreaking: return to the food traditions of generations past and see a reduction in many of our chronic health problems—especially those we have assumed were just "part of life." Our great-great-grandparents may not have known the word "lectin," but they knew how to prepare and enjoy food to minimize its deleterious effects. We can glean from their traditions and look to modern science as we hunt and gather our way to a reduced-lectin diet.

In this book, my goal is to blend ancient wisdom with the latest science to create delicious recipes that will help you reduce inflammation, lose weight, and prevent disease.

CHAPTER ONE

UNDERSTANDING LECTINS

One of the most famous, or should I say infamous, lectins is gluten. Today, we know it as the scourge of people with celiac disease. Even a crumb of wheat, barley, or rye can damage the lining of their small intestines and lead to malnutrition and disease. According to mounting research, it also affects individuals who don't have celiac disease but suffer from many of the same symptoms and get the cumbersome label, "non-celiac gluten sensitivity."

However, in the early 1900s, scientists didn't even consider gluten a possible culprit in celiac disease. They had observed it for centuries and documented its effects in medical journals, but its etiology was hardly understood. Popular treatments ranged from the bizarre—1 quart of mussels a day—to nearly impossible—200 bananas a week. And yet, no one thought to point the finger at gluten.

In the 1940s, a doctor in the Netherlands observed that the death rate for children with celiac disease plummeted from more than 35 percent to virtually zero during the Dutch famine when wheat flour was unavailable. The death rate returned to those staggeringly high levels when the famine was over and celiac children could eat bread again. He made the connection then between wheat and celiac.

It wasn't until the 1950s that scientists established a solid link between the gluten in wheat and celiac disease, and could finally confirm its presence by physical damage to the small intestine.

Why the history lesson? Because our knowledge of the effect of lectins is still at about that of the 1940s. Like the Dutch physician, some modern doctors have made the observations, such as Dr. Steven Gundry in his clinic and in his book, *The Plant Paradox*, along with many writers and lay scientists in the paleo community. But, the actual mechanism by which lectins make some people sick and overweight is poorly understood and poorly documented in scientific literature, with few credible clinical studies in humans about the effects of lectins.[1]

Nevertheless, we can see the effects of a low-lectin diet in our own bodies and in others who have adopted a low-lectin diet. We could wait another decade for clinical research to come along and support the protocol, or we could exclude the handful of foods that make us feel sick. This book offers the recipes to help you do that. But first, here's what science does tell us definitively about lectins.

What Are Lectins?

Lectins are proteins that bind to carbohydrates. They are found in virtually all living things—plants, animals, bacteria, and fungi— and have a myriad of biological functions within these organisms. In animals, they are involved in cell adhesion, cell reception, and immunity. In plants, they are involved in growth and possibly serve as a defense against predators.

Lectins are present in about 30 percent of our foods and are especially concentrated in the seeds and skin, or hull, of certain plants. They are also present in the animals we eat for food,

---

1   Most research that does enter the conversation on lectins focuses primarily on the effects of isolated lectins from raw legumes, which are clearly dangerous. But, these are rarely consumed, so those studies are somewhat irrelevant.

especially when those animals have consumed a high-lectin diet (grain fed and soybean fed).

The greatest concentrations of lectins in the human diet are found in legumes, grains, dairy, and nightshade plants, including tomatoes, potatoes, eggplant, and peppers. Hence, all of the recipes in this book exclude those foods entirely.

Some fruits that are usually thought of as vegetables contain low levels of lectins and can be problematic for some people. These foods include summer and winter squashes, cucumbers, and melons. I have used these ingredients sparingly in this book because most people find them tolerable.

What's Wrong with Lectins?

Lectins are thought to damage the lining of the small intestine, allowing small particles of food to escape into the bloodstream, where they provoke an immune response. This process is known as leaky gut syndrome and can contribute to autoimmune disorders.

According to an article published in the journal *Alternative Therapies in Health and Medicine* in 2015, lectins consumed in excess can cause nutrient deficiencies, disrupt digestion, and cause severe intestinal damage, all due to their carbohydrate-binding capabilities. An article published by Venezuelan researchers observed similar gut-disruptive effects, noting that lectins affect the turnover and loss of gut epithelial cells, damage the luminal membranes of the gut, interfere with nutrient digestion and absorption, stimulate shifts in the bacterial flora, and modulate the immune state of the digestive tract.

In plain language, lectins damage the cells that line the intestines, cause spaces to open between those cells, and prevent certain nutrients from being absorbed. Foods that contain lectins also contain protease inhibitors, which prevent enzymes from breaking down proteins.

Nevertheless, lectins don't affect everyone the same way, which is why so many people thrive on a diet that contains the staple foods listed above. Multiple theories exist to explain this reality. One theory is that individuals with dysfunctional enzymes are more susceptible to lectins in foods. Another theory is that lectins are only a problem for those who already have a permeable gut membrane, which could have occurred for a number of other factors. Finally, as I mentioned before, traditional preparation methods in global cultures minimize the damaging lectins.

What Not to Eat

The list of foods with the greatest concentration of lectins includes all grains, legumes, dairy products, and nightshade vegetables. It also includes some seeds and seed oils.

While some of the foods on the "what not to eat" list can be made safe through traditional preparation methods, this book provides recipes that are naturally free from these ingredients.

If you do opt to consume the foods on the no-go list, here are some preparation tips to reduce lectin:

- For fruit and vegetables, remove the peels and seeds.

- Choose refined grains, such as white rice, which is sometimes called a "safe starch."

- When cooking legumes, soak in unsalted water overnight. Rinse and drain. Cook in fresh, unsalted water at a high temperature (212°F) for at least one hour. A pressure cooker is ideal, but not necessary. A slow cooker does not get hot enough to destroy lectins.

All Grains

- Barley
- Buckwheat
- Corn
- Oats
- Rice
- Rye
- Wheat

All Legumes

- Beans
- Chickpeas
- Lentils
- Peanuts
- Soybeans*

* Fermented soy products, such as gluten-free soy sauce, are acceptable in small quantities because the fermentation process destroys most of the harmful lectins.

Some Vegetables and Fruit

- Bell peppers
- Chili peppers
- Eggplant
- Green beans
- Peas
- Potatoes
- Tomatoes

All Dairy

- Cheese
- Ice cream
- Milk
- Yogurt

Some Seeds

- Chia
- Pumpkin
- Quinoa
- Sunflower

Some Oils

- Canola oil
- Corn oil
- Soybean oil
- Sunflower oil

What to Eat

Good news, the list of foods you should eat is endless!

Fruit

All fruits are acceptable, including avocado and coconuts (coconut flour, coconut milk, coconut water, etc.). The exceptions are bell peppers, tomatoes, and eggplants, which are botanically considered fruits.

Vegetables

All vegetables except those listed on page 7 are acceptable.

Nuts

All nuts are acceptable in limited quantities, depending on your personal tolerance to them. While nuts do contain lectins, many individuals find them easier to digest than other food sources of lectins. To improve the digestibility of nuts, soak them in fresh water for up to eight hours, rinse, and drain. Allow to dry in a dehydrator or use immediately in a recipe. Nut flours are also acceptable, as well as products made with them.

Fish

All fish and shellfish are acceptable. Choose wild-caught, sustainably harvested fish whenever possible. Grain- and soy-fed farmed fish is not a good choice.

Poultry and Eggs

All types of poultry and eggs—chicken, turkey, duck, quail, etc.—are acceptable. Choose organic, pasture-raised poultry and eggs whenever possible to avoid lectins in grain-fed animals.

Meat

All types of meat—beef, pork, lamb, etc.—are acceptable. Choose organic, pasture-raised, or wild meat whenever possible to avoid lectins in grain-fed animals.

Fats

- Avocado oil
- Coconut oil
- Olive oil
- Sesame oil
- Lard
- Duck fat

Other

- Broth—If using store-bought, check label for peppers and tomatoes. Find broth recipes on pages 171 and 172.
- Coffee
- Dark chocolate (70% cacao or greater)
- Gluten-free soy sauce or coconut aminos
- Herbs—all
- Olives
- Pepper
- Salt
- Spices—all except chili pepper, paprika, cayenne, and those made from nightshade plants
- Vinegar—all except malt vinegar, which contains barley
- Wine

***

Nutrition facts are provided with all recipes and are listed per serving.

CHAPTER TWO

BREAKFASTS

Green Smoothie

My kids have grown up on this green smoothie, which is inspired by a version I found in a raw, vegan cookbook. It's a great way to start your day off with plenty of leafy greens and fruit. I love the flavor of cilantro in my green drinks, but it's not everyone's choice, so use parsley if you prefer. Serve with Vanilla Walnut Date Bars (page 12) for a complete breakfast.

Serves: 2   *Prep time:* 5 minutes   *Cook time:* none

Egg-Free, Vegan

1 orange, peeled

1 lime, peeled

1 cup frozen pineapple

1 small banana, frozen

2 cups roughly chopped kale leaves or spinach

½ cup roughly chopped cilantro

1 cup unsweetened Almond Milk (page 169)

Place all of the ingredients into a blender and puree until smooth.

Nutrition Facts: 175 Calories | Fat 2g | Protein 5g | Carbohydrates 40g | Fiber 8g

Vanilla Walnut Date Bars

I love whipping up a batch of these fruit and nut bars and wrapping them individually so I have a convenient breakfast or snack on the go. The variations are endless—see just a couple below. I take inspiration from the popular LÄRABARs available in most grocery stores. This version is much less expensive and completely customizable to your tastes.

Yield: 8 bars   *Prep time:* 5 minutes   *Cook time:* none

Egg-Free, Vegan

1¼ cups chopped walnuts

1 cup pitted, chopped dates

¼ teaspoon vanilla extract

⅛ teaspoon sea salt

1. Place the walnuts into a food processor and pulse until coarsely ground.

2. Add the dates to the food processor and pulse until the mixture is well blended and you can form it into a ball. Add the vanilla and sea salt and blend until fully incorporated.

3. Gather the contents of the food processor into a ball. On a cutting board, form into a flattened rectangle about ½-inch thick. Slice the rectangle into 8 bars. Wrap individually in parchment paper or plastic wrap, or store unwrapped in a covered container in the refrigerator for up to 1 week.

Nutrition Facts: 185 Calories | Fat 13g | Protein 3g | Carbohydrates 19g | Fiber 3g

Pumpkin Spice Date Bars: Replace the walnuts with pecans. Add 1 teaspoon pumpkin pie spice and 1 teaspoon orange juice.

Nutrition Facts: 192 Calories | Fat 14g | Protein 2g | Carbohydrates 19g | Fiber 4g

Chocolate Chip Cookie Dough Date Bars: Replace ½ cup of the walnuts with cashews. Add another ⅛ teaspoon sea salt. Add ¼ cup dairy-free dark chocolate chips; process in the food processor until they're just integrated and beginning to be chopped.

Nutrition Facts: 205 Calories | Fat 13g | Protein 4g | Carbohydrates 23g | Fiber 3g

Tropical Coconut Lime Date Bars: Replace the walnuts with 1 cup cashews and ½ cup toasted coconut. Add 1 tablespoon lime juice and the zest from 1 lime.

Nutrition Facts: 194 Calories | Fat 11g | Protein 4g | Carbohydrates 24g | Fiber 3g

Banana Nut Mousse

Creamy macadamia nuts and coconut milk are blended with bananas, maple syrup, and a hint of vanilla in this sweet treat that tastes more like dessert than breakfast! But, it's actually pretty good for you—complex carbohydrates and satisfying, healthy fats will keep you energized for hours!

Serves: 4   *Prep time:* 10 minutes, plus 30 minutes soaking time and 1 hour chilling time   *Cook time:* none

Egg-Free, Vegan

½ cup macadamia nuts, soaked in hot water for at least 30 minutes

2 ripe bananas, sliced, divided

1 cup full-fat coconut milk

2 tablespoons maple syrup, plus more to taste

2 teaspoons vanilla extract

1 teaspoon ground cinnamon

pinch sea salt

2 tablespoons coconut oil

¼ cup roughly chopped toasted pecans

1. Place the macadamia nuts, half of the bananas, coconut milk, maple syrup, vanilla, cinnamon, and sea salt into a blender. Puree until very smooth.

2. With the motor still running, slowly pour in the coconut oil.

3. Pour into individual serving cups and top with the remaining sliced banana and chopped pecans. Chill until ready to serve, about 1 hour.

Tip: I like to make these up the night before so they're ready to go for breakfast in the morning.

Nutrition Facts: 415 Calories | Fat 36g | Protein 3g | Carbohydrates 26g | Fiber 4g

Mixed Berry Parfait

When I gave up grains and dairy, one of the breakfasts I missed most was yogurt with fresh berries and granola. Eggs and bacon became redundant quickly. This cool, sweet treat answered my cravings. It combines fresh berries, creamy macadamia mousse, and crunchy toasted pecans.

Serves: 4   *Prep time:* 5 minutes   *Cook time:* none

Egg-Free, Vegan

4 cups assorted fresh berries, such as raspberries, blueberries, and strawberries

1 cup Sweet Vanilla Macadamia Mousse (page 170)

¼ cup toasted pecans

Layer the berries and macadamia mousse in a glass. Top with the toasted pecans.

Nutrition Facts: 380 Calories | Fat 19g | Protein 4g | Carbohydrates 27g | Fiber 11g

Apple Cinnamon Pancakes

These pancakes have all of the flavors of fall. They're delicious on brisk mornings when you have a little extra time to linger over breakfast and a steaming cup of coffee. For the best flavor, use Pink Lady or Granny Smith apples.

Serves: 4   *Prep time:* 10 minutes   *Cook time:* 20 minutes

Vegetarian

6 eggs	1 teaspoon baking soda
2 tablespoons maple syrup, plus more to serve	¼ teaspoon sea salt
	1 tablespoon ground cinnamon
¼ cup coconut milk	1 cup shredded peeled apple, from about 2 small apples
¼ cup coconut flour	
1 cup blanched almond flour	2 tablespoons coconut oil

1. Place the eggs, maple syrup, and coconut milk in a blender. Puree until smooth and the volume begins to increase.

2. Add the coconut flour, almond flour, baking soda, salt, and cinnamon. Puree until smooth, scraping down the sides as needed.

3. Squeeze some of the excess moisture from the shredded apple and add it to the blender. Pulse once or twice, just to integrate.

4. Heat a large skillet or griddle over medium heat. Melt some of the coconut oil and add pancake mixture to pan. Cook the pancakes for 3 to 4 minutes. Flip when the edges are set and bubbles appear near the center of the pancakes. Cook for another minute on the second side. Transfer to a serving platter.

5. Repeat until all of the batter is used up, adding more coconut oil as needed to grease the pan.

Tip: To shred the apples, peel and core them and then run through a food processor fitted with the grater attachment.

Nutrition Facts: 410 Calories | Fat 29g | Protein 17g | Carbohydrates 26g | Fiber 7g

Oven-Roasted Vegetables with Eggs

Oven-roasted vegetables with fried eggs are my favorite breakfast after a long morning of surfing. I suppose by then you could call it brunch, or even lunch. Whatever you call it, this meal supplies all of the complex carbohydrates, protein, and fat that I need to keep me energized and strong.

Serves: 4   *Prep time:* 10 minutes   *Cook time:* 25 minutes

Nut-Free, Vegetarian

4 sweet potatoes, sliced in ½-inch-thick pieces

1 fennel bulb, halved, cored, and sliced in ½-inch-thick wedges

2 zucchini, halved and sliced in ½-inch-thick pieces

1 red onion, halved and sliced in ½-inch-thick pieces

1 teaspoon minced fresh thyme

3 tablespoons extra-virgin olive oil, divided

4 eggs

sea salt, to taste

freshly ground pepper, to taste

1. Preheat the oven to 375°F.

2. Spread the sweet potatoes, fennel, zucchini, red onion, and thyme on a large rimmed baking sheet. Drizzle with 2 tablespoons of the olive oil and toss gently to coat the vegetables in oil. Season generously with salt and pepper.

3. Roast for 25 minutes, or until the vegetables are gently browned but not burned.

4. Meanwhile, heat a large skillet over medium-high heat until it is very hot. Add the remaining tablespoon of olive oil. Let it heat for 15 seconds.

5. Crack the eggs into the pan and cook until the whites are set and the yolk is still runny, 4 to 5 minutes.

6. Divide the roasted vegetables between serving plates and top with the fried eggs.

Nutrition Facts: 341 Calories | Fat 16g | Protein 10g | Carbohydrates 42g | Fiber 8g

Apple Sage Breakfast Sausage

Most commercial breakfast sausages contain nightshades and other unsuitable fillers. This sausage has all of the flavor without the lectin ingredients.

Serves: 4   *Prep time:* 5 minutes   *Cook time:* 10 minutes

Egg-Free, Nut-Free, Allergen-Free

1 pound ground pork	1 tablespoon minced fresh sage
½ cup minced peeled apples	½ teaspoon sea salt
1 shallot, minced	¼ teaspoon freshly ground pepper

1. Combine the ground pork with the apples, shallot, sage, salt, and pepper in a small mixing bowl.

2. Heat a large skillet over medium heat. Crumble the sausage mixture into the pan and saute for 10 minutes, until fully browned. Alternately, shape the mixture into 8 individual patties. Cook for 5 minutes on each side, until gently browned and cooked through.

Nutrition Facts: 348 Calories | Fat 24g | Protein 29g | Carbohydrates 3g | Fiber <1g

Sweet Potato Hash Browns

Sweet potatoes make just as good of hash browns as do traditional white potatoes. The trick is to avoid stirring them so they can get crisp on the outside and become tender and sweet on the inside.

Serves: 4   *Prep time:* 10 minutes   *Cook time:* 20 minutes

Egg-Free, Nut-Free, Allergen-Free, Vegan

> 4 medium sweet potatoes, peeled
>
> 2 tablespoons coconut oil
>
> sea salt, to taste

1. Grate the sweet potatoes using a food processor or box grater and thoroughly squeeze out excess moisture using your hands.

2. Heat the coconut oil in the cast-iron skillet over medium heat.

3. When the pan is hot, sprinkle the sweet potatoes into the pan and season with salt.

4. Cook for at least 10 minutes, until a brown crust forms on the bottom. Flip the sweet potatoes to brown on the other side, being careful not to stir too much. Cook for another 10 minutes, until gently browned. Serve immediately.

Nutrition Facts: 198 Calories | Fat 7g | Protein 2g | Carbohydrates 32g | Fiber 4g

Crepes with Strawberries and Macadamia Mousse

Decadent breakfasts don't have to be a thing of the past on a lectin-avoidance diet. These grain-free crepes are filled with Sweet Vanilla Macadamia Mousse.

Serves: 4   *Prep time:* 10 minutes   *Cook time:* 45 minutes

Vegetarian

8 teaspoons coconut oil, melted, divided

4 eggs

½ cup unsweetened Almond Milk (page 169)

1 teaspoon vanilla extract

2 tablespoons coconut flour

1 tablespoon tapioca starch

¼ teaspoon sea salt

1 cup Sweet Vanilla Macadamia Mousse (page 170)

2 cups sliced strawberries

1. Preheat the oven to 375°F. Coat the interior of an 8 x 8-inch baking dish with 1 teaspoon of coconut oil.

2. Combine the eggs, almond milk, and vanilla in a blender. Pulse once or twice. Add the coconut flour, tapioca starch, and sea salt. Blend until smooth, scraping down the sides as needed. Set the batter aside for 10 minutes to thicken.

3. Heat a large skillet over medium heat. Melt 1 teaspoon of the coconut oil in the pan. Pour 2 to 3 tablespoons of the crepe batter into the pan and tilt to spread. Cook for 1 to 2 minutes until set. Flip and cook for another 30 seconds. Transfer to a plate. Repeat with the remaining batter, using additional coconut oil as needed.

4. Fill each crepe with about 2 tablespoons of the macadamia mousse, then fold each crepe into a small burrito shape. Place them into the baking dish. Drizzle with the remaining 2

teaspoons of coconut oil and bake for 20 minutes, until the filling is heated through and the crepes begin to brown.

5. To serve, top with fresh strawberries.

Nutrition Facts: 464 Calories | Fat 41g | Protein 10g | Carbohydrates 20g | Fiber 6g

Chocolate Crepes with Raspberries and Macadamia Mousse: This makes a gorgeous Valentine's Day brunch or dessert. It is somewhat reminiscent of cannoli, with the cacao nibs in the macadamia mousse. Add ¼ cup cocoa powder and ¼ cup unsweetened almond milk to the crepe batter. Swap the strawberries for raspberries. Fold ¼ cup of cacao nibs into the macadamia mousse.

Nutrition Facts: 511 Calories | Fat 45g | Protein 12g | Carbohydrates 26g | Fiber 10g

Cinnamon Spice Granola

Unlike granola made with oats and tons of sugar, this one won't send your blood sugar into the stratosphere. Even better, it tastes amazing and will keep you full for hours. It reminds me of an oatmeal raisin cookie.

Serves: 7   *Prep time:* 5 minutes   *Cook time:* 19 minutes

Vegetarian

2 cups pecans	¼ teaspoon ground nutmeg
2 cups almonds	½ cup coconut oil, melted
2 cups walnuts	1 tablespoon vanilla extract
1 egg white	½ cup brown sugar
1 teaspoon ground cinnamon	½ teaspoon sea salt
¼ teaspoon ground ginger	1 cup packed raisins

1. Preheat the oven to 325°F.

2. Place the pecans, almonds, and walnuts in a food processor and blend until the mixture is coarsely ground.

3. In a blender, combine the egg white, cinnamon, ginger, nutmeg, coconut oil, vanilla, brown sugar, and sea salt. Blend until emulsified.

4. Pour the egg white mixture into the food processor with the nut mixture and pulse a few times, just until integrated.

5. Pour the mixture onto a sheet pan and flatten gently with a metal spatula.

6. Bake for 5 to 7 minutes. Stir the mixture and bake for another 5 to 7 minutes. Stir again and bake for a final 5 minutes, or until beginning to brown.

7. Allow the granola to cool completely on the pan, then stir in the raisins, transfer to an airtight container, and store.

Nutrition Facts: 497 Calories | Fat 46g | Protein 10g | Carbohydrates 25g | Fiber 7g

Chocolate Crunch Granola: Add ¼ cup of unsweetened cocoa powder and an additional ¼ teaspoon of sea salt to the granola. Omit the raisins and stir in ½ cup cocoa nibs after the granola has baked.

Nutrition Facts: 477 Calories | Fat 48g | Protein 11g | Carbohydrates 21g | Fiber 7g

Sausage, Mushroom, and Spinach Frittata

Frittatas work for breakfast, lunch, or dinner. They're perfectly versatile—see the delicious variations that follow—and provide a complete meal in just one pan. The trick is to keep the pan hot enough so that the eggs don't stick when you fry them.

Serves: 4   *Prep time:* 10 minutes   *Cook time:* 25 minutes

Nut-Free

8 ounces pork sausage, casings removed, crumbled

1 teaspoon olive oil

1 cup sliced mushrooms

1 shallot, halved and thinly sliced

1 cup roughly chopped spinach

8 eggs, whisked

sea salt, to taste

freshly ground pepper, to taste

1. Preheat the oven to 375°F.

2. Heat a large oven-proof skillet over medium heat. Cook the sausage until it is browned, about 5 minutes. Transfer it to a separate dish.

3. Add the olive oil to the pan. Sear the mushrooms for 5 minutes, until gently browned.

4. Add the shallot and spinach to the pan and cook until the spinach is wilted but has not lost its liquid, about 1 minute.

5. Return the sausage to the pan along with any accumulated juices. Season generously with salt and pepper.

6. Add the eggs to the pan and cook for 5 minutes. Transfer to the oven and cook for another 5 to 7 minutes, or until the eggs are just set.

Nutrition Facts: 390 Calories | Fat 30g | Protein 26g | Carbohydrates 2g | Fiber <1g

Bacon Avocado Frittata: Avocados might sound strange in a frittata, but they're surprisingly delicious and creamy. Swap the sausage for 4 strips of applewood-smoked bacon. Cook for 10 minutes. Skip the shallot, mushrooms, and spinach. Pour in the eggs and then arrange the slices from 1 large avocado in the center of the skillet. Cook for 5 minutes on the stove and 5 to 7 minutes in the oven.

Nutrition Facts: 256 Calories | Fat 20g | Protein 15g | Carbohydrates 5g | Fiber 3g

Sweet Potato, Mushroom, and Spinach Frittata: For a vegetarian frittata, swap the sausage for 2 cups Essential Roasted Sweet Potatoes (page 65). Add it to the pan after browning the mushrooms.

Nutrition Facts: 258 Calories | Fat 14g | Protein 14g | Carbohydrates 17g | Fiber 2g

Coffee Cake

This is my version of the classic Starbucks coffee cake. It has far less sugar and, like all of the recipes in this book, is gluten-free and dairy-free.

Serves: 12   *Prep time:* 10 minutes   *Cook time:* 30 minutes
Vegetarian

1 cup brown sugar	*Topping:*
½ cup palm shortening	¼ cup palm shortening
3 eggs	¼ cup brown sugar
1 tablespoon vanilla extract	¼ cup almond flour
2 cups blanched almond flour	1 tablespoon ground cinnamon
2 tablespoons coconut flour	¼ teaspoon sea salt
1 tablespoon ground cinnamon	
1 teaspoon sea salt	
1 teaspoon baking soda	

1. Preheat the oven to 350°F. Line the interior of an 8 x 8-inch baking dish with parchment paper.

2. Beat the brown sugar and shortening together in a large mixing bowl until thick and creamy.

3. Add the eggs and vanilla, and whisk until thoroughly emulsified.

4. Sift in the almond flour, coconut flour, cinnamon, sea salt, and baking soda.

5. Spread the batter in the prepared pan.

6. To make the topping, combine the palm shortening, brown sugar, almond flour, cinnamon, and sea salt. Crumble the mixture over the cake batter.

7. Bake for 30 minutes, or until a tester comes out clean.

Nutrition Facts: 310 Calories | Fat 25g | Protein 6g | Carbohydrates 26g | Fiber 3g

Sausage and Sweet Potato Strata

Savory pork sausage, thinly sliced sweet potatoes, and fresh thyme baked in a coconut milk and egg custard. This one-dish breakfast is great for preparing the night before so that all you need to do is bake it in the morning.

Serves: 8   *Prep time:* 10 minutes   *Cook time:* 55 minutes

Nut-Free

1 tablespoon coconut oil	1 teaspoon sea salt
16 ounces Apple Sage Breakfast Sausage (page 20) or another nightshade-free sausage	½ teaspoon freshly ground pepper
1 cup coconut milk	1 tablespoon minced fresh thyme
8 eggs, whisked	3 sweet potatoes, thinly sliced to about ⅛-inch thick

1. Preheat the oven to 375°F. Coat the interior of a 2-quart baking dish with the coconut oil.

2. Heat a large skillet over medium heat. Cook the sausage until gently browned and cooked through, about 5 minutes.

3. In a separate bowl, whisk the coconut milk, eggs, salt, pepper, and thyme.

4. Spread the sweet potato slices into the baking dish, allowing them to overlap slightly. Top with about ⅓ of the sausage. Pour ¼ of the coconut-egg mixture over the sausage.

5. Repeat the process, finishing with the remaining coconut milk. Cover the pan tightly with foil and bake for 40 minutes. Remove the foil and cook for another 10 minutes, until gently browned and bubbling.

Nutrition Facts: 363 Calories | Fat 24g | Protein 22g | Carbohydrates 14g | Fiber 2g

Winter Vegetable and Herb Strata

This recipe works as well for breakfast as it does for a simple dinner. Parsnip, turnip, fennel, and onion roast until caramelized before whisked eggs are poured into the dish to hold everything together. Slice into wedges. Serve with a drizzle of Garlic Aioli (page 162).

Serves: 4   *Prep time:* 5 minutes   *Cook time:* 40 to 50 minutes

Nut-Free, Vegetarian

2 parsnips, cut into 1-inch pieces

1 sweet potato, cut into 1-inch pieces

1 turnip, cut into 1-inch pieces

1 fennel bulb, trimmed and cut into 1-inch pieces

1 red onion, cut into 1-inch pieces

2 tablespoons minced fresh herbs, such as rosemary, thyme, and parsley

2 tablespoons extra-virgin olive oil

8 eggs, whisked

sea salt, to taste

freshly ground pepper, to taste

1. Preheat the oven to 400°F.

2. Place the parsnips, sweet potato, turnip, fennel, onion, and herbs into an 8 x 10-inch baking dish. Drizzle with the olive oil and season generously with salt and pepper.

3. Bake for 35 to 40 minutes, until the vegetables are deeply browned and soft.

4. Season the eggs with salt and pour into the baking dish. Bake for another 5 to 10 minutes, or until the eggs are just set. Allow to cool for 5 minutes before serving.

Nutrition Facts: 259 Calories | Fat 13g | Protein 15g | Carbohydrates 21g | Fiber 5g

Broccoli Egg Muffin Cups

These make the perfect breakfast when you're on the go. I like to make a big batch ahead of time and then just heat and serve when I'm on my way out the door. They're also customizable so each person gets just what they like. I use green onions here because they do not need to be cooked beforehand.

Yield: 12 muffins   *Prep time:* 10 minutes   *Cook time:* 15 to 18 minutes
Nut-Free

2 cups frozen broccoli florets, defrosted

4 slices (about ¼ cup) cooked bacon, crumbled

2 green onions, thinly sliced

12 eggs, whisked

½ teaspoon sea salt

¼ teaspoon freshly ground pepper

1. Preheat the oven to 350°F. Line a 12-cup muffin tin with parchment paper liners.

2. Divide the broccoli, bacon, and onions between the muffin cups.

3. Whisk the salt and pepper into the eggs and carefully pour the mixture into the muffin cups until they are nearly full.

4. Bake for 15 to 18 minutes, until the eggs are set.

Tip: Parchment paper liners really do make a difference here and are preferable to regular paper liners, which will adhere to the eggs.

Nutrition Facts: 93 Calories | Fat 6g | Protein 7g | Carbohydrates 1g | Fiber 1g

Dutch Babies

I developed this recipe while working on my book, *Cast Iron Paleo*, and it quickly became a staple breakfast. My kids request it often. Even on busy mornings, it is easy to whip up, pop into the oven, and bake while we get ready to head out the door.

Serves: 4   *Prep time:* 5 minutes   *Cook time:* 20 minutes

Vegetarian

½ cup unsweetened Almond Milk (page 169)

2 tablespoons maple syrup, plus more to serve

1 tablespoon vanilla extract

2 tablespoons coconut flour

⅓ cup tapioca starch

¼ teaspoon sea salt

1 dozen eggs

2 tablespoons coconut oil

1. Preheat the oven to 400°F.

2. Combine the almond milk, maple syrup, vanilla, coconut flour, tapioca starch, sea salt, and eggs in a blender. Puree until smooth, scraping down the sides as needed.

3. Heat a large cast-iron skillet, or another oven-proof skillet, over medium-high heat. When it is very hot, melt the coconut oil in the skillet.

4. Pour the egg mixture into the pan and transfer it to the oven. Bake for 20 minutes, or until golden and puffy. Serve with additional maple syrup.

Nutrition Facts: 326 Calories | Fat 22g | Protein 20g | Carbohydrates 12g | Fiber 2g

CHAPTER THREE

SNACKS AND SMALL BITES

Prosciutto-Wrapped Dates

I first tried prosciutto-wrapped dates at a little tapas bar in downtown Denver called the 9th Door. They were so addicting, I couldn't wait to return to the restaurant. Eventually we moved away and I knew I had to take that magical combination of sweet and salty flavors with me. They were surprisingly easy to recreate; I instantly felt silly for not making them sooner!

Serves: 4   *Prep time:* 10 minutes   *Cook time:* 15 to 18 minutes

Egg-Free

16 Medjool dates, pitted

16 Marcona almonds or blanched almonds

2 ounces Manchego cheese, cut into 16 small pieces

8 slices prosciutto, sliced in half lengthwise

1. Preheat the oven to 375°F. Line a sheet pan with parchment paper.

2. Place 1 almond and 1 small piece of Manchego into the center of each date.

3. Wrap each date tightly with the prosciutto and place seam-side down on the sheet pan.

4. Bake for 15 to 18 minutes, until the prosciutto begins to brown.

Tip: Manchego is a sheep's milk cheese and is tolerable to some people on a lectin-avoidance diet. If you don't do well with it, simply omit it from the recipe.

Nutrition Facts: 242 Calories | Fat 10g | Protein 9g | Carbohydrates 33g | Fiber 4g

Root Vegetable Latkes

Latkes are traditionally made with grated potato, but other root vegetables work equally well. Try parsnip, rutabaga, turnip, sweet potato, and even beets. Squeeze as much of the liquid from the grated vegetables as you can for maximum crispiness. Serve with Garlic Aioli (page 162).

Serves: 4 *Prep time:* 5 minutes *Cook time:* 9 minutes

Egg-Free, Nut-Free, Allergen-Free, Vegetarian

1 pound parsnips, turnips, or other root vegetables

2 tablespoons coconut flour

1 egg, whisked

1 tablespoon minced fresh rosemary

½ teaspoon sea salt

½ teaspoon freshly ground pepper

2 tablespoons canola oil or coconut oil

1. Grate the root vegetables using a box grater or a food processor fitted with the grater attachment.

2. Take a handful of the grated vegetables and, holding them over the sink, squeeze as much water from them as you can. Repeat with the remaining vegetables.

3. Preheat a large skillet over medium-high heat.

4. Place the grated vegetables into a bowl and toss gently to coat in the coconut flour. Add the egg, rosemary, salt, and pepper.

5. When the skillet is hot, add the oil and tilt to coat the pan. Scoop smallish portions of the grated vegetables into the pan and flatten gently with a spatula. Allow to sear on one side undisturbed for about 5 minutes, or until it forms a deep golden crust. Flip and sear for another 4 minutes on the second side. You may have to do this in batches to avoid crowding the pan.

Nutrition Facts: 130 Calories | Fat 9g | Protein 3g | Carbohydrates 11g | Fiber 4g

Rosemary Almond Crackers

These crackers satisfy the urge to snack on something crisp and are the perfect vehicle for dips and spreads. The versatility of these crackers lends itself well to other flavor combinations. Swap the rosemary for 1 tablespoon of nutritional yeast and 1 teaspoon of garlic powder for a savory cracker. Or, use another fresh herb, such as sage or thyme.

Serves: 8 (2 crackers per serving)   *Prep time:* 5 minutes   *Cook time:* 10 minutes

Egg-Free, Vegan

2 cups blanched almond flour

1 tablespoon minced fresh rosemary

¼ teaspoon sea salt

1 tablespoon olive oil

1 teaspoon maple syrup

2 to 3 tablespoons ice water, divided

1. Preheat the oven to 325°F.

2. Combine the almond flour, rosemary, and sea salt in a small bowl. Drizzle in the olive oil, maple syrup, and 1 tablespoon of ice water.

3. Stir just until the mixture comes together in a ball, adding more water a teaspoon at a time as needed.

4. Roll the dough between 2 sheets of parchment paper until very thin. Remove the top sheet of parchment and transfer the dough to a large baking sheet.

5. Cut the dough into 16 individual crackers.

6. Bake for 10 minutes, or until the crackers begin to brown around the edges.

7. Transfer to a cooling rack and cool for 10 minutes, or until completely cool, before serving or storing in a covered container.

Nutrition Facts: 177 Calories | Fat 16g | Protein 6g | Carbohydrates 7g | Fiber 3g

Roasted Parsnip Fries with Hazelnut Picada

Parsnips are a root vegetable with a creamy color and texture. They're shaped like carrots and have a mild flavor similar to but more muted than sweet potatoes, making them a perfect canvas for other flavors. In this recipe, I roast them until they're well caramelized and chewy, and top them with a simple picada of hazelnuts, parsley, and vinegar. Serve them with a simple pan-seared salmon or roasted chicken for a complete meal.

Serves: 4   *Prep time:* 5 minutes   *Cook time:* 35 to 45 minutes

Egg-Free, Vegan

4 parsnips, cut lengthwise into quarters

3 tablespoons olive oil

2 tablespoons roughly chopped, toasted hazelnuts

2 tablespoons minced fresh parsley

1 teaspoon sherry vinegar

sea salt, to taste

freshly ground pepper, to taste

1. Preheat the oven to 425°F. Line a sheet pan with parchment paper.

2. Place the parsnips on the sheet pan. Toss with the olive oil and season with salt and pepper.

3. Roast for 35 to 45 minutes, until deeply browned and soft.

4. Combine the hazelnuts and parsley in a mortar and pestle and bash gently until well combined but still crumbly. Season with salt and pepper. Stir in the vinegar just before serving.

5. Spread the parsnip fries onto a serving platter and top with the hazelnut picada.

Nutrition Facts: 204 Calories | Fat 11g | Protein 2g | Carbohydrates 27g | Fiber 6g

Coconut Shrimp with Mango Dipping Sauce

Ubiquitous on appetizer menus, this sweet and savory appetizer is often coated with wheat and paired with a chili dipping sauce. For a lower-lectin option, try these crispy, coconut-encrusted shrimp with a tangy mango dipping sauce.

Serves: 4   *Prep time:* 10 minutes   *Cook time:* 10 to 12 minutes

Nut-Free

1 teaspoon sea salt

1 teaspoon garlic powder

¼ cup coconut flour

2 egg whites

1 pound large shrimp, butterflied

1 cup shredded unsweetened coconut

1 cup cubed mango

2 tablespoons lime juice

1 teaspoon gluten-free soy sauce or coconut aminos

1 teaspoon minced fresh ginger

1. Preheat the oven to 425°F. Line a sheet pan with parchment paper.

2. Combine the salt, garlic powder, and coconut flour in a small bowl.

3. In a separate bowl, whisk the egg whites.

4. Dip each shrimp in the coconut flour mixture to coat thoroughly. Then dip it into the egg whites. Finally, dip each shrimp into the shredded coconut and place onto the baking sheet. Repeat until all of the shrimp have been coated in the coconut mixture.

5. Bake for 10 to 12 minutes until the coconut is gently browned and the shrimp are cooked through.

6. While the shrimp bake, combine the mango, lime juice, soy sauce, and ginger in a blender, and puree until smooth.

7. Serve the coconut shrimp with the mango sauce on the side.

Nutrition Facts: 319 Calories | Fat 16g | Protein 27g | Carbohydrates 19g | Fiber 6g

Asian Chicken Wings

Most chicken wing recipes are loaded with nightshades, such as peppers and tomatoes. This version takes the classic appetizer in a different direction with spicy ginger, savory toasted sesame oil, and tangy lime juice. Serve them with the Mixed Herb Salad with Ginger Lime Vinaigrette (page 50).

Serves: 6   *Prep time:* 5 minutes   *Cook time:* 30 minutes

Egg-Free, Nut-Free

4 cloves garlic

1 lime, zest and juice

¼ cup gluten-free soy sauce or coconut aminos

2 tablespoons minced ginger

1 tablespoon toasted sesame oil

½ teaspoon freshly ground pepper

2 pounds chicken wings

1. Preheat the oven to 425°F. Line a sheet pan with parchment paper.

2. Place the garlic, lime zest and juice, soy sauce, ginger, sesame oil, and pepper in a blender, and puree until smooth.

3. Pour the marinade over the chicken wings and toss gently to coat.

4. Spread the chicken wings onto the sheet pan and bake for 30 minutes, or until browned and crisp.

Tip: Prepare the marinade ahead of time and allow the chicken to marinate in the refrigerator for up to 8 hours.

Nutrition Facts: 276 Calories | Fat 8g | Protein 38g | Carbohydrates 2g | Fiber 0g

Essential Sweet Potato Avocado Toast

Avocado toast is all the rage, but on a grain-free diet, it's probably not something you even tempt yourself with. Sweet potatoes make the perfect stand-in for toast, and they are far more flavorful than bread. Here is the first of 4 versions of the savory snack. Double the portion size to make it a meal.

Serves: 4   *Prep time:* 5 minutes   *Cook time:* 30 minutes

Egg-Free, Nut-Free, Allergen-Free, Vegan

2 medium sweet potatoes, sliced in ⅛-inch slices

1 tablespoon canola oil or coconut oil

2 avocados, thinly sliced

1 teaspoon red wine vinegar

sea salt, to taste

freshly ground pepper, to taste

1. Preheat the oven to 375°F. Line a sheet pan with parchment paper.

2. Place the sweet potatoes in a small bowl and toss with the canola oil.

3. Spread the sweet potatoes out on the sheet pan and season with salt. Bake for 30 minutes, or until gently caramelized and shrunken.

4. When the sweet potatoes are done cooking, allow them to cool for about 5 minutes.

5. Place the sweet potato slices on a serving plate and top each with a few slices of avocado. Season with salt and pepper and a splash of the red wine vinegar. Serve immediately.

Nutrition Facts: 243 Calories | Fat 17g | Protein 3g | Carbohydrates 23g | Fiber 8g

Smoked Salmon Sweet Potato Avocado Toast

This avocado toast is similar to lox and cream cheese on bagels. It has the briny capers, salty smoked salmon, and spicy red onion. The avocado stands in beautifully for cream cheese.

Serves: 4   *Prep time:* 5 minutes   *Cook time:* 30 minutes

Egg-Free, Nut-Free

2 medium sweet potatoes, sliced to ⅛-inch slices

1 tablespoon canola oil or coconut oil

½ cup thinly sliced red onion

2 tablespoons red wine vinegar

2 avocados, thinly sliced

4 ounces lox or smoked salmon

2 tablespoons capers, drained

sea salt, to taste

freshly ground pepper, to taste

1. Preheat the oven to 375°F. Line a sheet pan with parchment paper.

2. Place the sweet potatoes in a small bowl and toss with the canola oil.

3. Spread the sweet potatoes out on the sheet pan and season with salt. Bake for 30 minutes, or until gently caramelized and shrunken.

4. While the sweet potatoes cook, place the onion in a bowl, season with sea salt, and pour the red wine vinegar over the top.

5. When the sweet potatoes are done cooking, allow them to cool for about 5 minutes.

6. Remove the red onion from the vinegar and shake off any excess.

7. Place the sweet potato slices on a serving plate and top each with a few slices of avocado, a piece of lox, a few pieces of

red onion, and a few capers. Season with salt and pepper. Serve immediately.

Nutrition Facts: 285 Calories | Fat 18g | Protein 8g | Carbohydrates 25g | Fiber 8g

Middle Eastern Sweet Potato Avocado Toast

If pita and hummus was one of your favorite snacks before you gave up grains and legumes, you'll love these sweet potato toasts. Za'atar is a Middle Eastern spice blend with thyme, sesame seeds, and ground sumac. It is naturally free of nightshades and is available in the spice aisle of many grocery stores, or online. You can also make your own.

Serves: 4   *Prep time:* 5 minutes   *Cook time:* 30 minutes

Egg-Free, Nut-Free, Allergen-Free, Vegan

2 medium sweet potatoes, sliced to ⅛-inch slices

1 tablespoon canola oil or coconut oil

1 tablespoon tahini

1 tablespoon lemon juice

1 tablespoon extra-virgin olive oil

2 avocados, thinly sliced

½ cup thinly sliced red onion

1 tablespoon Za'atar (page 178)

sea salt, to taste

1. Preheat the oven to 375°F. Line a sheet pan with parchment paper.

2. Place the sweet potatoes in a small bowl and toss with the canola oil.

3. Spread the sweet potatoes out on the sheet pan and season with salt. Bake for 30 minutes, or until gently caramelized and shrunken.

4. In a small bowl, whisk the tahini, lemon juice, and olive oil. Season to taste with salt.

5. When the sweet potatoes are done cooking, allow them to cool for about 5 minutes.

6. Place the sweet potato slices on a serving plate and top each with a few slices of avocado and a few pieces of red onion. Drizzle with the tahini dressing and top with a pinch of Za'atar. Serve immediately.

Nutrition Facts: 243 Calories | Fat 17g | Protein 3g | Carbohydrates 23g | Fiber 8g

Bacon and Chives Sweet Potato Avocado Toast

These savory bites make the perfect party snack. Smoky bacon and minced fresh chives taste like your favorite potato chip, only better.

Serves: 4   *Prep time:* 5 minutes   *Cook time:* 30 minutes

Egg-Free, Nut-Free, Allergen-Free

2 medium sweet potatoes, sliced to ⅛-inch slices

1 tablespoon canola oil or coconut oil

2 avocados, thinly sliced

4 slices bacon, cooked and crumbled

2 tablespoons minced fresh chives

sea salt, to taste

freshly ground pepper, to taste

1. Preheat the oven to 375°F. Line a sheet pan with parchment paper.

2. Place the sweet potatoes in a small bowl and toss with the canola oil.

3. Spread the sweet potatoes out on the sheet pan and season with salt. Bake for 30 minutes, or until gently caramelized and shrunken.

4. When the sweet potatoes are done cooking, allow them to cool for about 5 minutes.

5. Place the sweet potato slices on a serving plate and top each with a few slices of avocado, bacon, and chives. Season with salt and pepper, and serve immediately.

Nutrition Facts: 287 Calories | Fat 20g | Protein 6g | Carbohydrates 23g | Fiber 8g

Root Vegetable Chips

One of my favorite snacks from Trader Joe's is the Root Vegetable Chips. But, I prefer a baked, not deep-fried, snack, and these homemade veggie chips are ideal. They're loaded with fiber and antioxidants and are a cinch to make.

Serves: 4   *Prep time:* 5 minutes   *Cook time:* 15 minutes

Egg-Free, Nut-Free, Allergen-Free, Vegan

1 pound assorted root vegetables, such as beets, sweet potatoes, and turnips, sliced paper-thin

2 tablespoons canola oil or coconut oil, melted

sea salt, to taste

1. Preheat the oven to 350°F. Line a sheet pan with parchment paper.

2. Toss the root vegetables with the oil and spread them across the sheet pan so that they're in a single layer and not touching one another. You will have to do this in batches. Season with sea salt.

3. Bake for 15 minutes or until crisp and beginning to brown. Be careful not to burn them. Spread the chips onto a cooling rack and bake the remaining vegetables.

Tip: Use the largest sheet pan you have available so that the vegetables aren't crowded together. This will help them crisp up during baking.

Nutrition Facts: 157 Calories | Fat 7g | Protein 2g | Carbohydrates 23g | Fiber 3g

Grilled Mushrooms

These grilled mushrooms are one of my favorite side dishes to serve with grilled meat and fish. They cook easily along the sides of the grill while the main dish is cooking.

Serves: 4   *Prep time:* 5 minutes   *Cook time:* 5 to 7 minutes

Egg-Free, Nut-Free, Allergen-Free, Vegan

2 tablespoons fresh thyme leaves

¼ cup roughly chopped cilantro

1 shallot, roughly chopped

2 cloves garlic, minced

2 tablespoons sherry vinegar

¼ cup extra-virgin olive oil

¼ teaspoon sea salt

¼ teaspoon freshly ground pepper

1 pint cremini mushrooms

1. Preheat a grill to medium heat.

2. Combine the thyme, cilantro, shallot, garlic, sherry vinegar, olive oil, salt, and pepper in a blender, and puree until mostly smooth.

3. Thread the mushrooms onto bamboo or metal skewers. Brush them with the herb mixture. Grill for 5 to 7 minutes or until the mushrooms are tender but not charred.

Nutrition Facts: 142 Calories | Fat 14g | Protein 1 | Carbohydrates 4g | Fiber 1g

CHAPTER FOUR

SOUPS, SALADS, AND SIDES

Mixed Herb Salad with Ginger Lime Vinaigrette

Refreshing, tangy, and spicy, this side salad pairs well with fish and grilled meat. Any tender salad green such as spring mix or baby spinach will work for the salad greens.

Serves: 4   Prep time: 5 minutes   Cook time: none

Egg-Free, Nut-Free, Allergen-Free, Vegetarian

2 tablespoons lime juice

1 teaspoon minced ginger

2 tablespoons extra-virgin olive oil

1 teaspoon honey

4 cups mixed salad greens

2 cups mixed herbs, such as mint, basil, and cilantro

sea salt, to taste

freshly ground pepper, to taste

1. Whisk the lime juice, ginger, olive oil, and honey in a small bowl. Season generously with salt and pepper.

2. Add the mixed greens and herbs, and toss gently to mix. Serve immediately.

Tip: Remove mint leaves from the stems. The basil and cilantro stems are full of flavor; just discard the tough ends.

Nutrition Facts: 81 Calories | Fat 7g | Protein 1g | Carbohydrates 1g | Fiber 2g

Romaine Hearts with Creamy Scallion Dressing

The dressing on this salad is so good I could drink it from the jar, and it's perfect over whatever sturdy mixed greens you want to toss it with. I suggest romaine hearts here, but spinach and kale also work. Just don't use baby salad greens, which will not stand up to the weight of the dressing.

Serves: 4   *Prep time:* 5 minutes   *Cook time:* none

Egg-Free, Nut-Free, Allergen-Free, Vegan

½ bunch scallions (about 4), green parts only, diced

½ bunch parsley, tough stems removed

1 tablespoon fresh thyme leaves

½ tablespoon Dijon mustard

½ teaspoon sea salt

1 lemon, zest and juice

2 tablespoons white wine vinegar

¼ cup extra-virgin olive oil

2 romaine hearts, roughly chopped

1. Combine the scallions, parsley, thyme, Dijon mustard, salt, lemon zest and juice, white wine vinegar, and olive oil in a blender. Puree until smooth.

2. Place the romaine lettuce in a large bowl and pour the dressing over the greens. Toss gently to coat.

Nutrition Facts: 135 Calories | Fat 14g | Protein 2g | Carbohydrates 3g | Fiber 2g

Green Goddess Kale Salad

Most bottled green goddess dressing contains dairy. This version is mayonnaise-based for a low-lectin option. But, it still has all of the flavor of the original, thanks to fresh tarragon. For a vegetarian version, leave out the anchovy.

Serves: 4   *Prep time:* 5 minutes   *Cook time:* none

2 tablespoons minced fresh chives

¼ cup minced fresh parsley

2 tablespoons minced fresh tarragon

1 teaspoon minced garlic

1 tablespoon lemon juice

1 teaspoon anchovy paste (optional)

¼ cup mayonnaise

1 head lacinato kale, roughly chopped

1 teaspoon extra-virgin olive oil

¼ cup roughly chopped pistachios

sea salt, to taste

1. Combine the chives, parsley, tarragon, garlic, lemon juice, anchovy paste, if using, and mayonnaise in a blender. Puree until smooth, scraping down the sides as needed with a spatula.

2. Place the kale into a mixing bowl and season with salt. Drizzle with the olive oil and use your hands to massage the oil into the kale, until it is wilted. Divide the kale between serving plates and top with the green goddess dressing and a tablespoon of the pistachios.

Tip: I prefer to use an immersion blender for making the dressing because it is such a small amount. Alternately, double the dressing recipe and store half of it in a covered container in the refrigerator for up to 3 days.

Nutrition Facts: 218 Calories | Fat 16g | Protein 7g | Carbohydrates 17g | Fiber 6g

French Onion Soup

Onions are an underappreciated vegetable, but they really shine in this starter soup. It's naturally nightshade free, but definitely read the label on purchased beef broth to ensure it doesn't contain any other ingredients.

Serves: 4   *Prep time:* 10 minutes   *Cook time:* 80 minutes

Egg-Free, Nut-Free, Allergen-Free

2 tablespoons olive oil

3 yellow onions, halved and thinly sliced

¼ cup dry red wine

1 quart beef broth

1 sprig fresh thyme

1 sprig fresh rosemary

sea salt, to taste

1. In a large pot over medium heat, cook the onions in the olive oil with a generous pinch of salt. Cover and cook for 30 minutes.

2. Uncover and cook the onions until they are golden brown, about 30 minutes more.

3. Pour in the red wine, broth, thyme, and rosemary. Bring to a simmer and cook for 20 minutes. Remove the herbs.

Nutrition Facts: 125 Calories | Fat 6g | Protein 7g | Carbohydrates 9g | Fiber 2g

French Onion Soup with Chicken: If you love French onion soup as much as I do, transform it into a complete meal by adding chicken thighs. Just before adding the red wine and broth, push the onions to the side and add 1 pound of boneless, skinless chicken thighs, cut into 1-inch pieces. Brown on all sides and then add the wine, broth, and herbs. Simmer until the chicken is cooked through, about 5 minutes.

Nutrition Facts: 273 Calories | Fat 11g | Protein 32g | Carbohydrates 9g | Fiber 2g

Parsnip Bisque with Balsamic Red Onions

This silky pureed soup is the perfect started to a holiday meal. Parsnips are best after the first frost of the season has helped the root vegetable convert its starches into sugar. I use my own homemade vegetable broth in this recipe because it doesn't overshadow the parsnips, but use what you have on hand.

Serves: 4   *Prep time:* 10 minutes   *Cook time:* 30 minutes

Egg-Free, Nut-Free, Allergen-Free, Vegan

1½ tablespoons extra-virgin olive oil, divided

1 yellow onion, sliced

½ teaspoon minced fresh garlic

1 pound parsnips, peeled and roughly chopped

4 cups Vegetable Broth (page 172)

1 cup coconut milk

¾ teaspoon sea salt, divided

1 red onion, halved and very thinly sliced

½ teaspoon freshly ground pepper

1½ teaspoons minced fresh rosemary

1 tablespoon balsamic vinegar

1 tablespoon maple syrup

1. In a large pot, heat 1 tablespoon of the oil over medium heat. Add the yellow onion and cook until soft but not browned, about 8 minutes. Add the garlic and cook for another minute.

2. Add the parsnips, vegetable broth, and coconut milk to the pot, and bring to a simmer. Season with ½ teaspoon of the salt. Cover and cook for 20 minutes, until the parsnips are tender. Use an immersion blender to puree the soup until smooth. Alternatively, carefully transfer the soup in batches to a blender and puree. Cover the top of the blender lid with a towel and vent the lid to avoid splatters.

3. While the soup cooks, heat a skillet over high heat. When it is hot, add the remaining ½ tablespoon of oil. Tilt to coat the pan.

4. Add the ¼ teaspoon salt, red onion, pepper, and rosemary. Cook for 2 minutes, allowing the onion to brown slightly. Reduce the heat to medium-low and cook, stirring often, until the onion is very tender and beginning to caramelize. Stir in the balsamic vinegar and maple syrup.

5. To serve, divide the parsnip soup between serving bowls and top with 2 tablespoons of the caramelized onions.

Nutrition Facts: 288 Calories | Fat 17g | Protein 4g | Carbohydrates 34g | Fiber 6g

Smoky Sweet Potato Soup with Spinach

I made this soup for a church dinner in late October, when it makes sense to enjoy creamy, comforting soups. Although a heat wave had just rocked Santa Barbara, somehow the fall-themed soup still worked. The smoky flavors in the recipe come from smoked sea salt, but you can use liquid smoke or smoked black pepper if you prefer. If nightshades are not a problem for you, you can also add 1 teaspoon of smoked paprika.

Serves: 4   *Prep time:* 10 minutes   *Cook time:* 27 to 30 minutes

Egg-Free, Nut-Free, Allergen-Free

1 tablespoon coconut oil

1 yellow onion, diced

1 tablespoon minced fresh garlic

1 tablespoon ground cumin

4 medium sweet potatoes, peeled and diced

1 quart Chicken Broth (page 171) or Vegetable Broth (page 172)

½ teaspoon smoked sea salt

½ teaspoon freshly ground pepper

1 (15-ounce) can coconut milk

4 cups roughly chopped spinach

2 green onions, white and green parts, thinly sliced on a bias

1. Head the coconut oil in a large pot over medium-high heat.

2. Cook the onion for 9 minutes, or until golden and soft. A little bit of charring is okay.

3. Add the garlic and cumin, and cook for another minute.

4. Add the sweet potatoes, broth, salt, and pepper, and bring to a simmer. Cover and cook for 15 to 18 minutes or until the sweet potatoes are tender.

5. Stir in the coconut milk and heat for 1 minute.

6. Stir in the spinach and green onions, and cook for 1 minute, until the spinach is barely wilted.

Tip: You can use store-bought broth for this recipe, but read the nutrition labels. Many vegetable broths contain peppers and tomatoes.

Nutrition Facts: 373 Calories | Fat 23g | Protein 5g | Carbohydrates 40g | Fiber 5g

Creamy Celeriac Puree

Don't be intimidated by this knobby root vegetable, also called celery root. Once you peel away its tough exterior, the white flesh can be chopped and used just like potatoes to make a creamy, comforting side dish. The flavor is reminiscent of celery, but understated.

Serves: 4   *Prep time:* 5 minutes   *Cook time:* 30 minutes

Egg-Free, Nut-Free, Allergen-Free

1 (2-pound) celery root peeled and sliced into 1-inch pieces

1 sprig fresh thyme

1 clove garlic, smashed

1 (15-ounce) can full-fat coconut milk

2 cups Chicken Broth (page 171)

sea salt, to taste

1. Place the celery root in a large pot.

2. Add the thyme and garlic, and season liberally with salt.

3. Pour in the coconut milk and chicken broth and bring the mixture to a gentle simmer over medium heat. Cover, reduce the temperature to low, and cook until the celeriac is tender, about 30 minutes.

4. Remove the thyme sprig. Drain the celeriac, reserving 1 cup of the cooking liquid.

5. Use an immersion blender to puree the cooked celeriac, adding the reserved cooking liquid as desired until it reaches the desired consistency.

Nutrition Facts: 211 Calories | Fat 11g | Protein 5g | Carbohydrates 25g | Fiber 5g

Roasted Garlic Mashed Cauliflower

I am amazed by the power of cauliflower! It can be transformed into so many things. (I've even made frosting with it that my kids loved!) So, it's only natural that the white vegetable is the perfect stand-in for potatoes in this comfort-food side dish. The end result is creamy, pillowy, and far lower in calories.

Serves: 4   *Prep time:* 5 minutes   *Cook time:* 10 minutes

Egg-Free, Nut-Free, Allergen-Free

1 medium head cauliflower, broken into florets

½ cup Chicken Broth (page 171)

¼ cup coconut cream

1 tablespoon roasted garlic

½ teaspoon white wine vinegar

½ teaspoon sea salt

1. Place the cauliflower in a steamer basket set over simmering water in a large pot. Cover and steam for 10 minutes, or until the cauliflower is very tender.

2. Transfer the cooked cauliflower to a food processor along with the chicken broth, coconut cream, garlic, white wine vinegar, and sea salt. Blend until smooth. Serve immediately.

Nutrition Facts: 92 Calories | Fat 6g | Protein 3g | Carbohydrates 9g | Fiber 4g

Roasted Carrots with Carrot Top Pesto

I love buying bunches of carrots with the stems and lacy greens still attached, but it's such a shame to toss the tops into the compost bin. Instead, I combine them with fresh basil, garlic, and olive oil for a pungent pesto that livens up caramelized, roasted carrots.

Serves: 4   *Prep time:* 10 minutes   *Cook time:* 25 minutes

Egg-Free, Nut-Free, Allergen-Free, Vegan

1 bunch young carrots with 1-inch stems, greens reserved, and halved lengthwise

4 tablespoons extra-virgin olive oil, divided

½ cup fresh basil

1 large clove garlic

1 tablespoon minced red onion

2 tablespoons lemon juice

sea salt, to taste

freshly ground pepper, to taste

1. Preheat the oven to 375°F.

2. Spread the carrots out on a rimmed baking sheet and drizzle with 1 tablespoon of the olive oil. Season with salt. Roast for 25 minutes, or until tender and gently browned.

3. Meanwhile, combine the remaining 3 tablespoons of olive oil, basil, garlic, red onion, and lemon juice in a small food processor. Roughly chop the tender portions of the carrot tops until you have 1 packed cup of the greens, and add to food processor.

4. Pulse in the food processor until well combined. You can also use an immersion blender along with the measuring cup that accompanies it to blend the pesto. Season to taste with salt and freshly ground pepper.

5. Place the roasted carrots on a serving dish and drizzle with the pesto.

Tip: Leftover pesto can be stored in the refrigerator in a covered container for up to 3 days.

Nutrition Facts: 165 Calories | Fat 14g | Protein 1g | Carbohydrates 11g | Fiber 3g

Mashed Plantains with Bacon and Fennel

After trying mofongo at a Puerto Rican restaurant in Los Angeles, this is my favorite way to serve plantains. Make sure to pick medium-ripe plantains that still have a lot of green and no black spots on them. They develop a fruity funk when they're overripe. Also, the slightly underripe plantains are a great source of resistant starch, which feed your good gut bacteria.

Serves: 4   *Prep time:* 5 minutes   *Cook time:* 26 minutes

Egg-Free, Nut-Free, Allergen-Free

2 slices applewood-smoked bacon, sliced into lardons

½ cup thinly sliced fennel

1 teaspoon minced garlic

2 plantains, sliced into ½-inch-thick slices

cooking oil, as needed

sea salt, to taste

1. Cook the bacon pieces in a large skillet over medium heat until they render all of their fat, about 10 minutes. Use a slotted spoon to transfer the bacon to a separate dish.

2. Cook the fennel in the bacon fat until nearly soft, about 5 minutes. Add the garlic and cook for another minute. Transfer the fennel and garlic to the dish with the bacon.

3. Add additional oil to the pan if needed. Cook the plantains for 5 minutes on each side until browned and soft. Place them in a mortar and pestle and mash until they resemble mashed potatoes, although some chunks will still remain. Add the fennel and garlic, and mash until combined. Season to taste with salt.

Nutrition Facts: 199 Calories | Fat 5g | Protein 5g | Carbohydrates 37g | Fiber 3g

Sesame Ginger Rainbow Chard

Rainbow chard is perhaps one of the most beautiful garden vegetables. It is also remarkably easy to grow and to prepare. Here I sauté it with garlic, ginger, and toasted sesame oil and then add soy sauce, lime juice, and a touch of agave. The result is a versatile and flavorful side dish.

Serves: 4 *Prep time:* 5 minutes *Cook time:* 5 minutes

Egg-Free, Nut-Free, Allergen-Free, Vegan

1 tablespoon extra-virgin olive oil

1 teaspoon toasted sesame oil (optional)

1 bunch rainbow chard, stems diced and leaves cut in thin strips

1 teaspoon minced fresh garlic

1 teaspoon minced fresh ginger

2 tablespoons coconut aminos or gluten-free soy sauce

1 teaspoon agave or maple syrup

1 lime, juiced

1. Heat the olive oil and toasted sesame oil, if using, in a large, deep skillet over medium-high heat. When it is hot, add the chard, garlic, and ginger. Sauté for 3 minutes, until fragrant and wilted.

2. Meanwhile, whisk the coconut aminos, agave, and lime juice in a small jar. Pour this mixture over the chard and cook for 2 minutes, or until most of the liquid has evaporated from the pan. Serve immediately.

Tip: The oxalic acid in the chard and other greens can often make it astringent and give a chalky mouthfeel. Cooking neutralizes that flavor, but to be extra safe, blanch it in boiling water for 1 minute and then shock in an ice water bath. Pat dry and then proceed with the recipe.

Nutrition Facts: 87 Calories | Fat 5g | Protein 4g | Carbohydrates 10g | Fiber 4g

Pan-Roasted Apples and Crisp Sage

Fruit is a surprisingly delicious complement to savory food, especially these warm apples with crisp sage and red onion. Serve with Prosciutto-Wrapped Scallops (page 80) and Creamy Celeriac Puree (page 58) for a decadent fall dinner.

Serves: 2 to 4   *Prep time:* 5 minutes   *Cook time:* 12 minutes

Egg-Free, Nut-Free, Allergen-Free, Vegan

2 tablespoons extra-virgin olive oil

8 sage leaves

4 apples, peeled, cored, and sliced into wedges

1 red onion, halved and thinly sliced

¼ teaspoon ground cinnamon

¼ teaspoon minced fresh garlic

2 teaspoons lemon juice

sea salt, to taste

1. Heat the olive oil in a large skillet over high heat until hot but not smoking. Fry the sage leaves in the oil for about 5 seconds. Transfer to a paper towel–lined cooling rack to crisp up.

2. Reduce the heat to medium and add the apples and onion. Cook for about 10 minutes, until crisp-tender.

3. Add the cinnamon and garlic and cook for another 2 minutes. Season with the lemon juice and a generous pinch of salt.

4. Top with the crisp sage leaves to serve.

Nutrition Facts: 141 Calories | Fat 7g | Protein 1g | Carbohydrates 22g | Fiber 4g

Essential Roasted Sweet Potatoes

It's easy for a lectin-avoidance diet to become a low-carb diet. This starchy side dish is one of my kitchen staples and provides the complex carbohydrates to keep me full and energized. For a variation, you can cut the sweet potatoes into spears, like French fries, and bake as directed.

Serves: 4   *Prep time:* 5 minutes   *Cook time:* 30 to 35 minutes

Egg-Free, Nut-Free, Allergen-Free, Vegan

4 medium sweet potatoes, cut into 1-inch cubes

2 tablespoons coconut oil, melted

¼ teaspoon sea salt

1. Preheat the oven to 375°F.

2. Spread the sweet potatoes on a rimmed baking sheet. Drizzle with the coconut oil and toss gently to coat. Season with salt.

3. Bake for 30 to 35 minutes, or until the sweet potatoes are golden brown and slightly shrunken.

Tip: Make sure the sweet potatoes are spread out over the baking sheet so that they roast instead of steam.

Nutrition Facts: 196 Calories | Fat 7g | Protein 2g | Carbohydrates 32g | Fiber 4g

Sweet Potato Salad with Parsley and Pistachios

Serves: 4   *Prep time:* 5 minutes   *Cook time:* none

Egg-Free, Vegetarian

2 tablespoons extra-virgin olive oil

1 tablespoon sherry vinegar

1 teaspoon honey

¼ teaspoon sea salt

¼ cup minced fresh parsley

2 tablespoons minced shallot

¼ cup roughly chopped pistachios

1 recipe Essential Roasted Sweet Potatoes (page 65)

Combine all the ingredients except for the pistachios and sweet potatoes to make a dressing. Toss the roasted sweet potatoes in the dressing. Top with the pistachios.

Nutrition Facts: 300 Calories | Fat 17g | Protein 4g | Carbohydrates 34g | Fiber 5g

Roasted Brussels Sprouts

Roasting Brussels sprouts transforms them. They're smoky, caramelized, and tender, completely masking their stronger flavors that can turn off some people.

Serves: 4   *Prep time:* 5 minutes   *Cook time:* 30 minutes

Egg-Free, Nut-Free, Allergen-Free, Vegetarian

1 pound Brussels sprouts, outer leaves removed, halved

2 tablespoons extra-virgin olive oil, divided

sea salt, to taste

freshly ground pepper, to taste

1 tablespoon red wine vinegar

1 teaspoon minced fresh garlic

1 teaspoon honey

1. Preheat the oven to 375°F.

2. Spread the Brussels sprouts out on a rimmed baking sheet. Drizzle with 1 tablespoon of the oil and toss gently to coat. Season with salt and pepper

3. Bake for 30 minutes, or until the sprouts are deeply brown.

4. Meanwhile, whisk the remaining tablespoon of oil, red wine vinegar, garlic, and honey.

5. Toss the roasted Brussels sprouts with the dressing just before serving.

Nutrition Facts: 173 Calories | Fat 14g | Protein 4g | Carbohydrates 11g | Fiber 5g

Balsamic Roasted Brussels Sprouts: Swap the red wine vinegar and garlic for 2 tablespoons balsamic vinegar and 1 tablespoon honey. Pour the vinegar-honey mixture over the Brussels sprouts during the last 5 minutes of roasting. The flavors of balsamic vinegar intensify as they cook with the vegetables.

Nutrition Facts: 179 Calories | Fat 14g | Protein 4g | Carbohydrates 13g | Fiber 5g

Sweet Potato Holiday Dressing

Being on a restrictive diet during the holidays can be depressing, but with a few creative recipes, it doesn't have to be! This holiday dressing mimics the flavor and texture of the traditional Thanksgiving turkey stuffing.

Serves: 6   *Prep time:* 10 minutes   *Cook time:* 60 to 65 minutes

Egg-Free, Nut-Free, Allergen-Free

3 large white sweet potatoes, cut into ½-inch pieces

2 tablespoons minced fresh sage

2 tablespoons minced fresh parsley

1 tablespoon minced fresh thyme

3 tablespoons extra-virgin olive oil, divided

1 yellow onion, diced

3 celery stalks, diced

½ cup Chicken Broth (page 171)

sea salt, to taste

freshly ground pepper, to taste

1. Preheat the oven to 375°F.

2. Spread the sweet potatoes onto a large rimmed baking sheet and toss with the sage, parsley, and thyme. Drizzle with 2 tablespoons of oil and season generously with salt and pepper. Roast for 35 to 40 minutes, until gently browned and soft.

3. During the last 10 minutes of cooking, heat the remaining tablespoon of oil in a large skillet over medium heat. Cook the onion and celery until soft, about 10 minutes.

4. Remove the sweet potatoes from the oven and stir in the onion and celery. Remove 1 cup of this mixture and mash with a potato masher. Return it to the pan along with the chicken broth, stirring to mix.

5. Cover the pan tightly with foil and cook for another 15 minutes.

Tip: Complete steps 1 through 4 a day in advance. Cool, cover, and refrigerate the dressing, and then bake for 25 minutes just before serving.

Nutrition Facts: 153 Calories | Fat 7g | Protein 2g | Carbohydrates 21g | Fiber 4g

---

Roasted Cauliflower with Raisins and Pine Nuts

Liven up boring cauliflower by roasting it with olive oil and garlic and tossing with crunchy pine nuts and sweet raisins. This is one of my family's favorite appetizers.

Serves: 4   *Prep time:* 5 minutes   *Cook time:* 30 minutes

Egg-Free, Vegan

1 head cauliflower, broken into small florets

2 tablespoons extra-virgin olive oil

1 tablespoon minced fresh garlic

¼ cup minced fresh parsley

1 teaspoon lemon zest

¼ cup raisins

2 tablespoons red wine vinegar

sea salt, to taste

freshly ground pepper, to taste

1. Preheat the oven to 375°F.

2. Place the cauliflower, olive oil, garlic, parsley, and lemon zest in a bowl and toss to coat the cauliflower in the oil.

3. Spread the cauliflower florets out on a rimmed baking sheet. Season with salt and pepper

4. Bake for 30 minutes, or until the cauliflower is crisp and browned.

5. Toss the roasted cauliflower with the raisins and red wine vinegar, then top with the pine nuts.

Nutrition Facts: 175 Calories | Fat 12g | Protein 4g | Carbohydrates 17g | Fiber 5g

Maple Roasted Beets

The earthy flavor of beets is perfectly offset by sweet maple syrup and tangy red wine vinegar in this simple side dish. Maybe it's their brilliant color, but I think these beets belong on a holiday table. They're also delicious served chilled over mixed greens.

Serves: 4   *Prep time:* 10 minutes   *Cook time:* 35 to 40 minutes

Egg-Free, Nut-Free, Allergen-Free, Vegan

2 bunches beets, peeled

2 tablespoons extra-virgin olive oil

¼ cup maple syrup

¼ cup red wine vinegar

freshly ground pepper, to taste

sea salt, to taste

1. Preheat the oven to 375°F. Line a rimmed baking sheet with parchment paper.

2. Cut the beets into quarters. Place them onto the baking sheet and toss with the olive oil. Season with salt and pepper. Roast for 25 minutes, or until very tender.

3. Whisk the maple syrup and red wine vinegar together in a small glass measuring cup. Pour the mixture over the beets and continue roasting for another 10 to 15 minutes, until the glaze is thick and syrupy.

Tip: Use gloves when peeling the beets to avoid turning your hands a festive shade of fuchsia!

Nutrition Facts: 145 Calories | Fat 7g | Protein 1g | Carbohydrates 21g | Fiber 2g

CHAPTER FIVE

FISH AND SEAFOOD

Garlicky Steamed Clams in White Wine

I love ordering a big bowl of steamed clams in restaurants, but they often contain copious amounts of butter. This version has all of the savory flavors of the restaurant appetizer without the dairy.

Serves: 4   *Prep time:* 10 minutes   *Cook time:* 17 minutes

Egg-Free, Nut-Free

2 tablespoons extra-virgin olive oil

1 small yellow onion, minced

1 tablespoon minced fresh garlic

½ cup dry white wine

2 cups Chicken Broth (page 171)

2 pounds fresh clams, scrubbed and debearded

2 thyme sprigs

sea salt, to taste

freshly ground pepper, to taste

¼ cup minced fresh parsley

juice from ½ lemon

1. Heat the olive oil in a large pot over medium heat. Cook the onion and garlic for 5 minutes, until they begin to soften.

2. Add the white wine and cook for about 2 minutes to allow some of the alcohol to cook off.

3. Add the chicken broth, clams, and thyme sprigs. Season with salt and pepper, and give everything a good toss.

4. Cover and simmer gently until the clams have all steamed open, up to 10 minutes. Remove the thyme stems. Garnish with the fresh parsley and lemon juice.

Nutrition Facts: 476 Calories | Fat 17g | Protein 54g | Carbohydrates 19g | Fiber 0g

Steamed Mussels in Tarragon Coconut Broth

Mussels are my favorite shellfish. When they're perfectly cooked, they're tender, succulent, and brimming with the subtle flavors of the sea. Play off their silky texture with a creamy coconut and tarragon broth.

Serves: 4   *Prep time:* 10 minutes   *Cook time:* 17 minutes

Egg-Free, Nut-Free

1 tablespoon coconut oil

2 shallots, halved and thinly sliced lengthwise

1 teaspoon minced fresh garlic

¼ cup dry white wine

1 cup full-fat coconut milk

2 cups Chicken Broth (page 171)

2 pounds fresh mussels, scrubbed and debearded

2 tarragon sprigs, leaves removed and roughly chopped, stems reserved

sea salt, to taste

freshly ground pepper, to taste

1. Heat the coconut oil in a large pot over medium heat. Cook the shallots and garlic for 5 minutes, until they begin to soften.

2. Add the white wine and cook for about 2 minutes to allow some of the alcohol to cook off.

3. Add the coconut milk, chicken broth, mussels, and tarragon stems. Season with salt and pepper, and give everything a good toss.

4. Cover and simmer gently until the mussels have all steamed open, up to 10 minutes. Remove the tarragon stems. Garnish with the fresh tarragon leaves.

Tip: Wait until just before you cook the mussels to scrub them and remove the stringy "beards" that emerge from the shells.

Nutrition Facts: 534 Calories | Fat 24g | Protein 55g | Carbohydrates 21g | Fiber 0g

Crab Cakes

Old Bay Seasoning is a typical addition to crab cakes. Unfortunately, it contains nightshades. These crab cakes use a homemade Seafood Seasoning Blend (page 179) that's spicy, grassy, and complements the crab beautifully.

Serves: 4   *Prep time:* 5 minutes   *Cook time:* 15 minutes

½ cup mayonnaise

1 egg white, beaten

¼ cup almond flour

2 tablespoons coconut flour

1 tablespoon Seafood Seasoning Blend (page 179)

½ teaspoon sea salt

2 cloves garlic, minced

1 scallion, minced

1 pound lump crab meat

1–2 tablespoons coconut oil

½ cup Garlic Aioli (page 162)

1. Whisk together the mayonnaise, egg white, almond flour, coconut flour, Seafood Seasoning Blend, salt, garlic, and scallion. Fold in the crab meat gently until all of the ingredients are thoroughly integrated, without breaking up the pieces of crab.

2. Form the mixture into six 1-inch-thick cakes and set in the refrigerator for at least 1 hour.

3. Heat a large skillet over medium-high heat. Add the coconut oil and tilt to coat the pan.

4. Sear the crab cakes for 5 to 7 minutes on each side, or until golden brown and hot all the way through.

5. Serve crab cakes with a drizzle of garlic aioli each.

Nutrition Facts: 481 Calories | Fat 38g | Protein 28g | Carbohydrates 5g | Fiber 2g

Hazelnut-Crusted Halibut

I grew up in the Pacific Northwest and didn't realize how essential hazel-, nuts were to the local cuisine until I left. Fortunately, Oregon hazelnuts are available in stores or online. I prefer to purchase roasted hazelnuts, but see the tip below for how to roast them at home.

Serves: 4   *Prep time:* 10 minutes   *Cook time:* 5 to 6 minutes

Egg-Free

½ cup roasted hazelnuts

1 teaspoon garlic powder

½ teaspoon sea salt

½ teaspoon freshly ground pepper

4 (6-ounce) halibut filets

2 tablespoons coconut oil

1. Place the hazelnuts in a spice grinder or small food processor and blend until finely ground. Stop before the hazelnuts start releasing their oils.

2. Add the garlic powder, sea salt, and pepper to the blender and pulse once or twice, just to combine.

3. Spread the hazelnut mixture out in a shallow dish. Coat the halibut filets in the hazelnut mixture and set aside.

4. Heat a large skillet over medium-high heat until very hot. Add the coconut oil, tilting to coat the bottom of the pan.

5. Sear the halibut for 2 to 3 minutes on each side, longer if the filets are very thick. The fish is done when it is opaque all the way through and flakes easily with a fork.

Tip: To roast the hazelnuts, preheat the oven to 400°F. Spread the hazelnuts on a rimmed baking sheet and roast for 10 to 15 minutes, or until golden brown and fragrant. Allow them to cool briefly and then rub off the papery skins with a clean towel.

Nutrition Facts: 402 Calories | Fat 22g | Protein 48g | Carbohydrates 3g | Fiber 2g

Pistachio-Parsley Crusted Halibut: Use shelled ground pistachios in place of the hazelnuts, along with 2 tablespoons minced fresh parsley. Prepare the halibut as directed on previous page.

Nutrition Facts: 382 Calories | Fat 19g | Protein 49g | Carbohydrates 4g | Fiber 2g

Provençal Tuna

I usually pan-sear tuna, but slow roasting it in the oven with olive oil, herbs, garlic, and red onion yields a succulent, tender fish. It is also easier to avoid overcooking it than it is on the stovetop because even a few extra seconds on the stove can toughen the meaty fish. The amount of olive oil in this recipe might seem extravagant—and it is—but most of it gets poured off at the end, so you're not actually eating as much as the recipe calls for.

Serves: 4   *Prep time:* 5 minutes   *Cook time:* 12 to 15 minutes

Egg-Free, Nut-Free

2 pounds ahi tuna, cut into 1- to 2-inch pieces

2 sprigs fresh rosemary

4 sprigs fresh thyme

6 cloves garlic, smashed

½ small red onion, thinly sliced

1 cup extra-virgin olive oil

sea salt, to taste

freshly ground pepper, to taste

1. Preheat the oven to 325°F.

2. Spread the tuna in a single layer in a small baking dish or cast-iron skillet.

3. Season the fish generously with salt and pepper. Sprinkle the rosemary and thyme over the tuna. Tuck the garlic and onion evenly among the fish.

4. Pour the olive oil over the fish until it is just covered.

5. Cover the dish tightly with foil. Bake for 12 minutes. Remove the pan from the oven and allow the tuna to rest in the hot oil for 10 minutes. It will continue cooking. Serve warm.

Tip: This recipe pairs well with Roasted Carrots with Carrot Top Pesto (page 60).

Nutrition Facts: 302 Calories | Fat 10g | Protein 50g | Carbohydrates 8g | Fiber 0g

Pan-Seared Scallops with Wilted Spinach

Scallops have a silky texture and mild flavor—a good seafood choice if you're not a "fish person." They're also easy to prepare. The trick is to pat the scallops completely dry with paper towels before cooking and to heat up the pan until it's almost smoking hot before adding the oil. This results in a gorgeous brown sear that locks in all of those delicious juices. Spinach is just one option for a side dish—it's quick and healthy. You could also swap it for the Sesame Ginger Rainbow Chard (page 63).

Serves: 2 to 4   *Prep time:* 10 minutes   *Cook time:* 6 minutes

Egg-Free, Nut-Free

1 tablespoon extra-virgin olive oil

1 pound sea scallops (less than 15 per pound)

6 cups baby spinach

1 teaspoon garlic

1 tablespoon lemon juice

sea salt, to taste

freshly ground pepper, to taste

1. Preheat a large skillet over high heat until it is very hot. Add the olive oil and tilt to coat the pan. It should thin immediately but not smoke.

2. While the pan heats, pat the scallops completely dry with paper towels. Just before placing them in the pan, season generously with salt and pepper on one side.

3. Reduce the heat to medium-high. Place the scallops seasoned-side down into the hot pan and cook undisturbed for 2 minutes. Just before turning, season the scallops again with salt and pepper. Flip and cook for another 2 minutes on the second side. Transfer them to a serving dish.

4. Add the spinach and garlic to the pan and cook for 2 minutes, or until bright green and just wilted. Sprinkle with the lemon juice and serve alongside the scallops.

Nutrition Facts: 284 Calories | Fat 9g | Protein 41g | Carbohydrates 9g | Fiber 2g

Prosciutto-Wrapped Scallops

Smooth, buttery prosciutto matches the scallops' silky texture and infuses the shellfish with flavor. The recipe works best if you use large diver scallops. They're more expensive, so I tend to serve this on special occasions only. The dish is delicious with Pan-Roasted Apples and Crisp Sage (page 64).

Serves: 2   *Prep time:* 10 minutes   *Cook time:* 6 minutes

Egg-Free, Nut-Free

1 pound sea scallops (less than 15 per pound)

7 to 8 slices prosciutto, sliced in half lengthwise

1 tablespoon extra-virgin olive oil

sea salt, to taste

freshly ground pepper, to taste

1. Pat the scallops dry thoroughly with paper towels. Take a strip of prosciutto and wrap it around each one.

2. Preheat a large skillet over high heat until it is very hot. Add the olive oil and tilt to coat the pan. It should thin immediately but not smoke.

3. Just before placing the scallops in the pan, season generously with salt and pepper on one side.

4. Reduce the heat to medium-high. Place the scallops seasoned-side down into the hot pan and cook undisturbed for 2 to 3 minutes, until well browned. Just before turning, season the scallops again with salt and pepper. Flip and cook for another 2 to 3 minutes on the second side until well browned and hot all the way through. Transfer them to a serving dish.

Tip: The prosciutto should stay secured around each scallop. If not, secure it with a toothpick.

Nutrition Facts: 296 Calories | Fat 11g | Protein 41g | Carbohydrates 6g | Fiber 0g

Sesame-Crusted Ahi Tuna

This is a staple at Asian-fusion restaurants in Seattle and Portland, where I grew up. Fortunately, it's a cinch to make and doesn't require any fancy ingredients—so you can bring the gourmet experience right into your kitchen! Really amp up the nutty sesame flavor with toasted sesame oil. Serve with a simple Mixed Herb Salad with Ginger Lime Vinaigrette (page 50) and steamed white rice.

Serves: 4 *Prep time:* 5 minutes *Cook time:* 6 minutes
Egg-Free, Nut-Free

4 (6-ounce) ahi tuna steaks	1 tablespoon canola oil
½ cup sesame seeds	sea salt, to taste
1 teaspoon toasted sesame oil	freshly ground pepper, to taste

1. Pat the tuna steaks mostly dry with paper towels. Season generously with salt and pepper.

2. Spread the sesame seeds in a shallow dish and press the tuna steaks into them so they are coated on all sides.

3. Preheat a large skillet over medium-high heat until it is very hot. Add the sesame and canola oils and tilt to coat the pan. It should thin immediately but not smoke.

4. Sear the tuna for 1 minute on each side (for rare), until a thick brown crust forms but the tuna is still a deep pink in the center, but not cold. Serve immediately.

Tip: For the best quality, purchase frozen, vacuum-packed ahi tuna. Anything in the "fresh" case is often just defrosted. Instead, defrost the frozen fish just before you intend to cook it.

Nutrition Facts: 324 Calories | Fat 16g | Protein 41g | Carbohydrates 10g | Fiber 2g

Salmon Cakes

Canned salmon might not have the most alluring ring to it, but it is surprisingly flavorful and convenient for whipping up these salmon cakes. Choose wild salmon for the best nutrition. Serve with Green Goddess Kale Salad (page 52) for a complete meal.

Serves: 4 *Prep time:* 10 minutes *Cook time:* 28 minutes
Nut-Free

1 cup diced, peeled sweet potato	¼ teaspoon sea salt
1 egg	¼ teaspoon freshly ground pepper
2 green onions, minced	1 (16-ounce) can wild salmon
2 tablespoons coconut flour	2 tablespoons coconut oil

1. Place the sweet potato in a steamer basket fitted into a pot of simmering water. Cover and steam for 10 minutes or until just tender.

2. Place the sweet potato into a bowl and mash with a fork. Add the egg, green onions, coconut flour, salt, and pepper, and stir to mix. Stir in the salmon.

3. Form the mixture into 8 small cakes. Allow to rest for at least 10 minutes to let the coconut flour absorb some of the moisture.

4. Heat a large skillet over medium-high heat. When it is hot, add the coconut oil. Tilt to coat the pan.

5. Cook the salmon cakes in two batches for about 4 minutes on each side, until deeply browned.

Tip: If the salmon cakes are too loose, add another tablespoon of coconut flour.

Nutrition Facts: 289 Calories | Fat 16g | Protein 25g | Carbohydrates 11g | Fiber 3g

Tuna Burgers: These are perfect for days when you're cleaning out your pantry and have a few spare cans of solid tuna. Just don't use the soupy "chunk" tuna. Replace the salmon with solid tuna and add ¼ cup minced fresh celery to the burgers. Serve with butter lettuce leaves for a "bun" and a generous schmear of mayonnaise.

Nutrition Facts: 388 Calories | Fat 27g | Protein 25g | Carbohydrates 12g | Fiber 3g

Pine Nut–Crusted Salmon with Broccolini

Delicate basil and pungent garlic complement the earthy flavors of the salmon and toasted pine nuts in this one-pan dish. There is no need to toast the pine nuts separately because they will toast while the salmon cooks.

Serves: 4   *Prep time:* 10 minutes   *Cook time:* 9 minutes

Egg-Free

1 cup fresh basil

2 cloves garlic, minced, divided

1 teaspoon lemon juice

¼ cup plus 1 tablespoon extra-virgin olive oil, divided

1 bunch broccolini

1½-pound salmon filet

¼ cup finely ground pine nuts

sea salt, to taste

freshly ground pepper, to taste

1. Place the basil, half the minced garlic, lemon juice, and ¼ cup of olive oil into a blender or the cup of an immersion blender. Puree until smooth. Set aside.

2. Heat a large skillet over medium-high heat. Add the remaining 1 tablespoon of the olive oil. Sauté the broccolini for 5 minutes, until crisp-tender. During the last 30 seconds of cooking, add the remaining minced garlic to the pan. Transfer the broccolini to serving plates.

3. Pat the salmon dry with paper towels and season generously with salt and pepper. Coat it in the ground pine nuts.

4. Add additional oil to the pan if needed. Sear the salmon for 2 minutes on each side, until still deep pink in the center but beginning to flake with a fork.

5. To serve, drizzle the pesto over the salmon and broccolini.

Nutrition Facts: 484 Calories | Fat 33g | Protein 39g | Carbohydrates 10g | Fiber 6g

Garlic Shrimp Fettuccine

Serves: 2   *Prep time:* 10 minutes   *Cook time:* 5 minutes

2 tablespoons extra-virgin olive oil

12 ounces large shrimp, peeled and deveined

1 tablespoon minced fresh garlic

2 tablespoons fresh lemon juice

1 recipe Grain-Free Fettuccine (page 180) or Cappello's gluten-free fettuccine

2 tablespoons minced fresh parsley

sea salt, to taste

freshly ground pepper, to taste

1. Bring a large pot of salted water to a boil.

2. While the water heats, heat the oil in a large skillet over medium-high heat. Sauté the shrimp until nearly cooked through, about 4 minutes. Add the garlic and cook for another minute, being careful not to burn. Season generously with salt, pepper, and lemon juice. Remove the shrimp pan from the heat.

2. Cook the pasta for 90 seconds. Drain and add to the pan of cooked shrimp. Sprinkle with fresh parsley before serving.

Nutrition Facts: 549 Calories | Fat 28g | Protein 43g | Carbohydrates 32g | Fiber 2g

Pesto Shrimp Fettuccine: Reduce the olive oil to just 1 tablespoon and swap the garlic and parsley in this recipe for 1 cup of Pesto (page 163). Add it to the pan after adding the cooked pasta. Toss briefly and then remove from the heat.

Nutrition Facts: 714 Calories | Fat 44g | Protein 46g | Carbohydrates 37g | Fiber 6g

Bok Choy, Mushroom, and Shrimp Stir Fry

This stir fry is definitely more than the sum of its parts. Make sure to get the pan really hot before frying the bok choy to get a good sear on it. This recipe calls for 12 heads of baby bok choy, which are about 3 inches long and can be found in farmer's markets. If you're purchasing the palm-sized "baby" bok choy sold in most supermarkets, you'll only need 4 heads. Serve with steamed white rice for a complete meal.

Serves: 4   *Prep time:* 10 minutes   *Cook time:* 15 minutes

Egg-Free, Nut-Free

2 tablespoons coconut oil, divided

1 pound large shrimp, peeled and deveined

1 teaspoon toasted sesame oil

12 heads baby bok choy, halved

1 cup roughly chopped shiitake mushrooms

1 tablespoon minced garlic

1 tablespoon minced ginger

4 green onions, thinly sliced

¼ cup gluten-free soy sauce or coconut aminos

½ cup chicken broth

1 lime, juiced

1 teaspoon honey or agave

1 tablespoon arrowroot powder

1. Heat 1 tablespoon of coconut oil in a large skillet over medium-high heat. Sauté the shrimp until just cooked through, about 5 minutes. Set aside.

2. Wipe the pan clean with a paper towel and then return it to the medium-high heat. When it is very hot, add the remaining tablespoon of coconut oil and the toasted sesame oil.

3. When the oil shimmers, place the bok choy cut-side down into the pan. The oil will pop and spit, so use a frying screen. Cook the bok choy for 3 to 4 minutes, until deeply browned. Turn it over to sear on the other side for another 3 minutes.

4. Add the mushrooms, garlic, ginger, and green onions to the pan. Cook for 2 minutes, or until fragrant.

5. Whisk the soy sauce, chicken broth, lime juice, honey, and arrowroot powder in a large glass measuring cup. Pour this mixture into the pan and return the shrimp and any accumulated juices to the pan. Cook for 1 to 2 minutes, until just thickened.

Tip: If you cannot find fresh shiitake mushrooms, place 1 ounce of dried shiitake mushrooms in 1 cup of very hot water to soften, about 10 minutes. Drain and roughly chop the mushrooms.

Nutrition Facts: 219 Calories | Fat 9g | Protein 27g | Carbohydrates 7g | Fiber 1g

Green Bean, Leek, and Shrimp Stir Fry: Swap the bok choy and mushrooms for 1 pound trimmed French green beans and 1 thinly sliced leek. Cook the green beans for 6 to 8 minutes until crisp-tender. Add the leek in step 4 along with the garlic and ginger.

Nutrition Facts: 260 Calories | Fat 10g | Protein 28g | Carbohydrates 17g | Fiber 5g

Grilled Mahi Mahi with Pineapple Salsa

Mahi mahi was the first fish I cooked after moving out of my parents' house to go to college. Some friends and I picked the firm white fish because it had a meaty texture and was unlikely to fall through the grill grates. You can also use swordfish in this recipe.

Serves: 4   *Prep time:* 10 minutes   *Cook time:* 5 minutes

Egg-Free, Nut-Free

1 cup diced fresh pineapple	2 tablespoons fresh lime juice
1 mango, diced	4 (6-ounce) mahi mahi steaks
¼ cup minced fresh cilantro	1 tablespoon coconut oil
¼ cup minced red onion	sea salt, to taste
1 clove garlic, minced	freshly ground pepper, to taste

1. To prepare the salsa, combine the pineapple, mango, cilantro, onion, garlic, and lime juice. Season with salt and pepper. Set aside to allow the flavors to come together.

2. Preheat a grill or grill pan to medium-high heat. Pat the mahi mahi steaks dry with paper towels. Coat them in the coconut oil and season with salt and pepper.

3. Grill the mahi mahi for about 5 minutes on each side, until the fish flakes easily with a fork. Serve the grilled fish with the fruit salsa.

Nutrition Facts: 270 Calories | Fat 6g | Protein 41g | Carbohydrates 15g | Fiber 2g

Grilled Mahi Mahi Fish Tacos with Pineapple Salsa: Prepare the mahi mahi and pineapple salsa as directed. Divide between 8 grain-free tortillas, such as Siete Cassava and Coconut Tortillas or Julian Bakery Paleo Wraps. Top each taco with 2 tablespoons shredded cabbage (1 cup total) and 1 tablespoon Garlic Aioli (page 162).

Nutrition Facts: 511 Calories | Fat 25g | Protein 41g | Carbohydrates 40g | Fiber 5g

Smoked Salmon and Celeriac Casserole

Casseroles have a 1950s ring to them, but this creamy, smoky, and rich seafood dish gets an updated twist with smoked salmon, sliced celeriac, and fresh dill. Serve with a glass of bone dry white wine. Alternately, this makes a lovely brunch dish.

Serves: 4   *Prep time:* 15 minutes   *Cook time:* 1 hour

Nut-Free

2 tablespoons coconut oil, divided

1 onion, minced

1 cup coconut milk

4 eggs

¾ teaspoon sea salt, divided

½ teaspoon freshly ground pepper

1 (1½-pound) celeriac, peeled and sliced ⅛-inch thick

1 bunch fresh dill, minced

1 pound smoked salmon

1. Preheat the oven to 375°F. Coat the interior of a 2-quart baking dish with 1 tablespoon of oil.

2. Heat a large skillet over medium heat. Add the remaining tablespoon of the coconut oil and cook the onion with ¼ teaspoon salt until soft, about 10 minutes. Set aside.

3. In a separate bowl, whisk the coconut milk, eggs, ½ teaspoon salt, and pepper.

4. Spread the celeriac slices into the baking dish, allowing them to overlap slightly. Top with about ⅓ of the cooked onions and ⅓ of the fresh dill. Top with about ⅓ of the smoked salmon. Pour in about ¼ of the coconut egg mixture.

5. Repeat the process, layering the celeriac, onion, dill, salmon, and coconut milk. Complete the casserole with a layer of celeriac and top with the remaining coconut milk. Cover the pan tightly with foil and bake for 40 minutes. Remove the foil

and cook for another 10 minutes, until gently browned and bubbling.

Tip: To peel the celeriac, slice off each end. Stand the root vegetable on one of the cut ends and slice away the woody exterior to reveal the white flesh inside.

Nutrition Facts: 491 Calories | Fat 30g | Protein 33g | Carbohydrates 22g | Fiber 4g

Balsamic Honey Cod

Liven up basic cod with this flavorful marinade made with honey and balsamic vinegar. Serve with Balsamic Roasted Brussels Sprouts (page 67).

Serves: 4   *Prep time:* 5 minutes   *Cook time:* 15 minutes

Egg-Free, Nut-Free

1 teaspoon coconut oil

4 (6-ounce) cod filets

½ teaspoon sea salt

¼ teaspoon freshly ground black pepper

¼ cup balsamic vinegar

2 tablespoons honey

2 tablespoons minced shallots

1. Preheat the oven to 425°F. Coat the interior of a glass baking dish with oil.

2. Pat the cod filets dry with paper towels, place them into the baking dish, and season with the salt and pepper.

3. Whisk the balsamic vinegar, honey, and shallots together in a separate dish. Pour half of the mixture over the cod, turning to coat.

4. Bake for 10 minutes. Brush with the remaining glaze and bake for another 5 minutes, or until the fish flakes easily with a fork.

Tip: To cook the cod and Brussels sprouts at the same time, cook the sprouts on the bottom rack, closest to the element. This will help them to caramelize. Stir once or twice during the cooking process to prevent them from burning.

Nutrition Facts: 232 Calories | Fat 3g | Protein 38g | Carbohydrates 12g | Fiber 0g

CHAPTER SIX

POULTRY

Tarragon Honey Chicken with Butter Lettuce

Tarragon has a sweet, spicy flavor reminiscent of anise. In this recipe, it subtly infuses a honey Dijon vinaigrette used as a dressing for the lettuce and a marinade for the chicken.

Serves: 4   *Prep time:* 10 minutes plus 10 minutes to 8 hours to marinate   *Cook time:* 20 minutes

Egg-Free, Nut-Free, Allergen-Free

2 tablespoons honey

2 tablespoons lemon juice

1 tablespoon Dijon mustard

2 tablespoons minced fresh tarragon

2 tablespoons minced shallots

¼ cup extra-virgin olive oil

½ teaspoon sea salt

¼ teaspoon freshly ground pepper

8 boneless, skinless chicken thighs, about 2 pounds

2 heads butter lettuce, hand torn

1. Preheat the oven to 425°F.

2. Whisk the honey, lemon juice, mustard, tarragon, shallots, olive oil, salt, and pepper together. Place the chicken in a baking dish and pour half of the marinade over it. Allow to soak in the marinade for at least 10 minutes, or up to 8 hours in the refrigerator.

3. Place the chicken into the oven and bake for 20 minutes, or until cooked through. Shred the chicken into bite-size pieces with a fork.

4. Toss the butter lettuce with the remaining vinaigrette and divide between serving plates. Place the cooked chicken on top of the lettuce.

Tip: Never use marinade that has touched raw meat as a salad dressing. If you have excess on the chicken, cook it first before using.

Nutrition Facts: 332 Calories | Fat 19g | Protein 29g | Carbohydrates 11 | Fiber 1g

Rosemary Chicken Bacon Salad

This tasty entrée salad has it all—smoky bacon, seared chicken, fresh herbs, creamy avocado, and sweet cranberries all drenched in a tangy, bacon-infused dressing.

Serves: 4   *Prep time:* 10 minutes   *Cook time:* 15 minutes

Egg-Free, Nut-Free, Allergen-Free

4 slices applewood-smoked bacon

1 pound chicken breast tenders

1 tablespoon minced fresh rosemary

2 tablespoons white wine vinegar

1 tablespoon honey or maple syrup

1 teaspoon Dijon mustard

2 tablespoons extra-virgin olive oil

8 cups mixed greens

1 avocado, thinly sliced

¼ cup dried cranberries (optional)

sea salt, to taste

freshly ground pepper, to taste

1. In a large skillet, cook the bacon over low heat until it renders all of its fat, about 10 minutes. Transfer the cooked bacon to a separate dish.

2. Remove 1 tablespoon of the bacon fat to a small jar, and set aside.

3. Season the chicken with salt, pepper, and the rosemary. Sear on each side until well browned and cooked through, about 5 minutes.

4. Add the white wine vinegar, honey, mustard, and olive oil to the jar with the bacon fat. Season with salt and pepper. Cover tightly with a lid and shake to emulsify.

5. Place the salad greens into a large bowl and add the dressing. Toss gently to coat the greens in the dressing.

6. To assemble the salad, divide the greens between serving plates. Top with chicken tenders, sliced avocado, the cooked bacon, and cranberries, if using.

Nutrition Facts: 354 Calories | Fat 19g | Protein 30g | Carbohydrates 17g | Fiber 5g

Classic Cobb Salad: For fewer carbs and a little more protein, transform this into a classic cobb salad—minus the cheese—with just a few swaps. Skip the rosemary, honey, and cranberries and add 1 crumbled hardboiled egg to each salad.

Nutrition Facts: 387 Calories | Fat 24g | Protein 37g | Carbohydrates 7g | Fiber 5g

Creamy Chicken Thighs with Mushrooms and Port

Pan-seared chicken thighs with browned cremini mushrooms and a creamy port reduction are an elegant comfort food. They're delicious served with Creamy Celeriac Puree (page 58).

Serves: 4   *Prep time:* 5 minutes   *Cook time:* 15 minutes

Egg-Free, Nut-Free, Allergen-Free

2 tablespoons extra-virgin olive oil, divided

8 boneless, skinless chicken thighs (about 2 pounds)

1 cup thinly sliced cremini mushrooms

2 tablespoons minced shallots

¼ cup ruby port

⅓ cup coconut milk

sea salt, to taste

freshly ground pepper, to taste

1. Heat a large skillet over medium-high heat. When it is hot, add 1 tablespoon of the olive oil.

2. Pat the chicken thighs dry with paper towels and season generously with salt and pepper. Pan sear the chicken for 2 to 3 minutes on each side, until just cooked through. Transfer the chicken to a separate dish.

3. Return the pan to the heat and add the remaining tablespoon of oil. When it is hot, add the mushrooms to the pan and cook until well-browned on each side; about 5 minutes total. Push the mushrooms to the side of the pan.

4. Add the shallots to the pan and cook for 2 minutes, until fragrant.

5. Add the port to the pan and simmer to reduce for 2 to 3 minutes. Add the coconut milk and bring to a simmer.

6. Return the chicken and any accumulated juices to the pan and cook until the chicken is heated through, about 1 more minute.

Nutrition Facts: 290 Calories | Fat 16g | Protein 28g | Carbohydrates 3g | Fiber 0g

Creamy Chicken Thighs with Creamy Mushrooms and Garlic: Swap the shallots for 1 tablespoon minced garlic and 1 teaspoon minced rosemary. Add ¼ cup dry white wine in place of the port.

Nutrition Facts: 290 Calories | Fat 16g | Protein 28g | Carbohydrates 3g | Fiber 0g

Oven-Roasted Garlic Herb Chicken

Preparing your chicken "spatchcock" allows it to cook more evenly and browns more of the skin for an especially tasty bird. You can have your butcher do this for you, or follow the instructions in the tip. I prefer to season chicken gently by rubbing with garlic instead of using a garlic paste, which has a tendency to turn bitter if browned.

Serves: 4 *Prep time:* 10 minutes *Cook time:* 45 to 60 minutes

Egg-Free, Nut-Free, Allergen-Free

1 whole chicken, with skin (about 3 to 4 pounds)

1 clove garlic, halved

2 tablespoons extra-virgin olive oil

1 tablespoon minced fresh parsley

1 tablespoon minced fresh rosemary

1 tablespoon minced fresh thyme

sea salt, to taste

freshly ground pepper, to taste

1. Preheat the oven to 400°F.

2. Season the open cavity of the chicken with salt and pepper. Place the chicken onto the sheet pan with the cut-side down, spreading out the legs. Press down between the breasts to flatten the chicken. Dry thoroughly with paper towels.

3. Rub the chicken skin and underside with the cut side of the garlic, then drizzle with oil. Season with salt and pepper and the parsley, rosemary, and thyme.

4. Bake for 45 to 60 minutes, or until the chicken is cooked through and reaches an internal temperature of 155°F. It will continue cooking after it comes out of the oven and reach an internal temperature of 165°F.

Tip: To prepare the chicken, place it in a clean kitchen sink with the cavity facing up and the backbone closest to you. Use a serrated knife or kitchen shears and cut down one side of the backbone, slicing through the ribs. Carefully cut down the other side to remove the backbone. Reserve it for another use, such as making stock.

Nutrition Facts: 434 Calories | Fat 32g | Protein 34g | Carbohydrates 1g | Fiber 0g

Chicken and Sweet Potato Harvest Bowl

This recipe came about when I had plenty of Thanksgiving leftovers in my refrigerator and wanted a delicious, easy way to use them up that didn't taste like the same meal over and over again. If you're preparing this recipe any other time of the year—when whole turkeys are not filling the grocery store shelves—use a precooked rotisserie chicken or prepare the Oven-Roasted Garlic Herb Chicken (page 100). The time estimate is deceivingly short because it is really a recipe of assembly and calls for so many other recipes.

Serves: 4   *Prep time:* 10 minutes   *Cook time:* none

Egg-Free

2 tablespoons balsamic vinegar

1 tablespoon maple syrup

½ tablespoon extra-virgin olive oil

1 tablespoon minced shallots

8 cups shredded kale

2 cups shredded cooked chicken or turkey, preferably dark meat

1 recipe Balsamic Roasted Brussels Sprouts (page 67)

1 recipe Essential Roasted Sweet Potatoes (page 65)

½ cup Mulled Wine Cranberry Sauce (page 175)

½ cup Maple Spiced Pecans (page 176)

sea salt, to taste

freshly ground pepper, to taste

1. Whisk the balsamic vinegar, maple syrup, olive oil, and shallots in a large bowl. Season with salt and pepper. Add the kale to the bowl and toss gently to coat.

2. Divide the dressed kale between serving bowls. Top with chicken, Brussels sprouts, sweet potatoes, cranberry sauce, and walnuts.

Nutrition Facts: 739 Calories | Fat 39g | Protein 30g | Carbohydrates 77g | Fiber 16g

Cilantro Ginger Chicken

Spicy ginger, savory garlic, and grassy cilantro permeate this simple one-pan chicken meal. I'm partial to dark meat, so I've used leg quarters in this recipe. This cut includes both the leg and the thigh, and one of these should be an ample serving for one person.

Serves: 4   *Prep time:* 5 minutes, plus at least 1 hour to marinate   *Cook time:* 40 to 45 minutes

Egg-Free, Nut-Free, Allergen-Free

8 cloves garlic

1 tablespoon minced fresh ginger

½ cup roughly chopped fresh cilantro

2 tablespoons lime juice

¼ cup extra-virgin olive oil

½ teaspoon sea salt

½ teaspoon freshly ground pepper

4 (10- to 12-ounce) chicken leg quarters

1. Combine the garlic, ginger, cilantro, lime juice, olive oil, sea salt, and pepper in a blender and puree until mostly smooth.

2. Place the chicken in a zip-top bag or non-reactive dish and pour the marinade over the chicken, lifting up the skin gently to let the marinade get underneath and soak into the meat. Cover and refrigerate for at least 1 hour or up to 8 hours.

3. Preheat the oven to 400°F. Also heat a large cast-iron skillet over medium-high heat.

4. Remove the chicken from the marinade and shake off any excess.

5. When the skillet is hot, place the chicken skin-side down into the pan and sear until a golden-brown crust forms, about 5 minutes. Flip the chicken and transfer the pan to the oven. Bake for 35 to 40 minutes, or until the chicken is cooked through.

Nutrition Facts: 648 Calories | Fat 52g | Protein 46g | Carbohydrates 0g | Fiber 0g

Pan-Seared Chicken and Wine Reduction

The simplicity of this recipe belies its delicious flavors and texture. A red wine pan sauce picks up all of the juicy bits of the cooked chicken and a hint of garlic and soaks into the quickly sautéed zucchini. It pairs well with Creamy Celeriac Puree (page 58).

Serves: 4   *Prep time:* 10 minutes   *Cook time:* 15 to 17 minutes

Egg-Free, Nut-Free, Allergen-Free

4 boneless, skinless chicken breasts, pounded to ½-inch thickness

2 tablespoons extra-virgin olive oil, divided

2 medium zucchinis, quartered lengthwise and cut into ½-inch pieces

1 clove garlic, minced

½ cup dry red wine, such as Merlot

1 teaspoon minced fresh thyme

sea salt, to taste

freshly ground pepper, to taste

1. Heat a large skillet over medium-high heat. Pat the chicken breasts very dry with paper towels. Season generously with salt and pepper.

2. Pour 1 tablespoon of the olive oil into the pan and tilt to coat the pan. Allow the oil to heat up for up to 30 seconds. Place the chicken into the pan and sear for 3 to 4 minutes without disturbing it.

3. Flip the chicken and cook on the other side for 2 to 3 minutes, or until the chicken is cooked through. Transfer the chicken to a warmed dish, cover, and set aside.

4. Add the remaining tablespoon of oil to the skillet and allow it to get hot.

5. Sauté the zucchini for about 4 minutes, or until well browned but not soft. Add the garlic to the pan and cook for another minute.

6. Transfer the zucchini to the dish with the chicken.

7. Return the pan to the heat and add the red wine and thyme. Simmer gently until reduced by about half, about 5 minutes.

8. Divide the chicken and zucchini between serving plates and drizzle with the red wine pan sauce. Serve immediately.

Tip: To make the zucchini easier to digest and avoid lectins, slice away the inner core of each zucchini quarter to remove any seeds.

Nutrition Facts: 367 Calories | Fat 13g | Protein 54g | Carbohydrates 5g | Fiber 2g

Chicken Pot Pie

There's something so comforting about pies. Breaking through the tender, flaky crust into a hearty stew or sweet filling just does it for me! Fortunately, it's easy as, well, pie to make a yummy, grain-free pie crust. The trick is not to overwork the dough, or it will be tough.

Serves: 6   *Prep time:* 15 minutes   *Cook time:* 1 hour

3 tablespoons extra-virgin olive oil, divided

2 cups blanched almond flour

2 tablespoons coconut flour

½ teaspoon sea salt, plus more to taste

¼ cup palm shortening

1 egg

1 to 2 tablespoons ice water

2 pounds chicken thighs, cut into 1-inch pieces

1 yellow onion, minced

4 carrots, diced

2 celery stalks, minced

1 large sweet potato, peeled and cut into ½-inch dice

3 tablespoons tapioca starch

1 cup Chicken Broth (page 171)

1 tablespoon minced fresh thyme

1 teaspoon minced fresh rosemary

freshly ground pepper, to taste

1. Preheat the oven to 375°F. Coat the interior of six 2-cup ramekins with 1 tablespoon of the oil.

2. To make the crust, place the almond flour, coconut flour, and ½ teaspoon sea salt in a food processor, and pulse a few times. Add the shortening, egg, and 1 tablespoon of the ice water. Pulse a few times, just until integrated. It should form a ball and pull away from the sides. If not, add the remaining tablespoon of water 1 teaspoon at a time as needed. Set the dough aside.

3. To make the filling, heat a large skillet over medium-high heat. Add the remaining 2 tablespoons of oil and tilt the pan to coat.

4. Pat the chicken dry with paper towels and season with salt and pepper. Cook in the skillet, browning on all sides, for about 10 minutes total. Transfer to a separate dish.

5. Reduce the heat to medium and add the onion, carrots, and celery. Cook for 5 minutes, until somewhat softened. Add the sweet potato and cook for another 5 minutes.

6. Add the tapioca starch to the pan and stir to mix until it is nearly dissolved. Add the chicken broth, thyme, rosemary, and cooked chicken along with any accumulated juices. Bring to a simmer then remove from the heat.

7. Divide the filling between the ramekins.

8. Roll the dough between two sheets of parchment paper until it is about ⅛ inch thick. Using another ramekin, trace a circle with a sharp knife. Fit the crust on top of one of the pot pies and press it in around the edges to prevent the filling from bubbling out. Repeat with the remaining dough and pot pies. Make one or two slits in the center of each pot pie to allow steam to escape.

9. Place the ramekins on a rimmed baking sheet and bake for 40 minutes. Allow to cool for 15 minutes before serving.

Nutrition Facts: 542 Calories | Fat 39g | Protein 29g | Carbohydrates 25g | Fiber 8g

Moroccan Chicken

My friend Anna introduced me to this recipe many years ago, and it has captivated me ever since. Fresh citrus and spices infuse the chicken with flavor, and almonds, olives, and apricots make a flavorful sauce on the side. If possible, use Marcona almonds for this recipe.

Serves: 4   *Prep time:* 5 minutes   *Cook time:* 45 minutes

Egg-Free

½ lemon, thinly sliced

½ orange, thinly sliced

1 whole (3- to 4-pound) chicken

2 tablespoons extra-virgin olive oil

1 tablespoon powdered ginger

1 teaspoon ground cumin

1 teaspoon ground cinnamon

½ cup Chicken Broth (page 171)

1 cup assorted olives

½ cup dried apricots, halved

½ cup roasted almonds

sea salt, to taste

freshly ground pepper, to taste

1. Preheat the oven to 425°F.

2. Wedge the lemon and orange slices under the skin of the chicken. Coat the exterior of the chicken with the olive oil.

3. Combine the ginger, cumin, cinnamon, salt, and pepper in a small dish. Season the chicken all over with this mixture.

4. Roast the chicken in a large roasting pan for 30 minutes. Remove the pan from the oven, and baste the chicken with the pan juices.

5. Add the broth, olives, apricots, and almonds.

6. Continue roasting for another 15 minutes until the chicken is cooked through.

7. Place the whole chicken on a serving dish and spoon the almond mixture around it. Serve family style.

Nutrition Facts: 415 Calories | Fat 23g | Protein 35g | Carbohydrates 16g | Fiber 3g

Creamy Chicken Fettuccine Alfredo

Sometimes cuddling up with a big bowl of creamy pasta and binge-watching Netflix is just what you need to brighten a chilly winter evening. In this recipe, I use coconut milk, cashews, and roasted garlic for the sauce, instead of the traditional wheat-thickened cream sauce.

Serves: 4   *Prep time:* 10 minutes   *Cook time:* 9 minutes

Egg-Free

1 tablespoon extra-virgin olive oil	1 teaspoon fresh thyme
16 ounces chicken tenders	¾ teaspoon sea salt
½ cup cashews, soaked in boiling water for 30 minutes, drained	1 recipe Grain-Free Fettuccine (page 180) or Cappello's gluten-free fettuccine
1 cup coconut milk	freshly ground pepper, to taste
1 head roasted garlic	

1. Heat the oil in a large skillet over medium-high heat. Sauté the chicken until cooked through, about 5 minutes. Set aside.

2. To make the sauce, combine the cashews, coconut milk, roasted garlic, and thyme in a blender. Puree until very smooth. Add the sauce to the pan with the chicken and bring to a simmer. Cook for 2 minutes. Season with freshly ground pepper.

3. Meanwhile, bring a large pot of salted water to a boil. Cook the pasta for 90 seconds. Drain, reserving ½ cup of the pasta cooking liquid, and add the pasta to the pan with the chicken. Give everything a good toss before serving, adding some of the pasta cooking liquid to loosen the sauce if desired.

Nutrition Facts: 421 Calories | Fat 21g | Protein 33g | Carbohydrates 25g | Fiber 1g

Bacon Kumquat Roasted Game Hens

Kumquats sound exotic, but once I saw them growing by the side of the road—and picked more than I could possibly eat—and I realized that they're very similar to other citrus fruits, especially mandarin oranges. The primary difference is that the peel of kumquats is sweet and the flesh is sour. They form the basis of this sweet and sour glaze that will liven up game hens or, if you prefer, a whole roasted chicken.

Serves: 4   *Prep time:* 10 minutes   *Cook time:* 45 to 50 minutes

Egg-Free, Nut-Free, Allergen-Free

4 strips applewood-smoked bacon, cut into ½-inch pieces

4 Cornish game hens

1 cup fresh-squeezed orange juice

1 cup sliced kumquats

1 tablespoon honey

1 tablespoon sherry vinegar

sea salt, to taste

freshly ground pepper, to taste

1. Preheat the oven to 375°F.

2. In a large skillet, cook the bacon over low heat until it renders all of its fat, about 10 minutes. Transfer the cooked bacon to a separate dish. Reserve the bacon fat.

3. Meanwhile, pat the game hens dry with paper towels and season generously with salt and pepper. Coat them in 1 tablespoon of the rendered bacon fat, discarding all the rest of the fat from the pan. Roast the game hens for 25 minutes in a shallow baking dish.

4. Meanwhile, add the orange juice and kumquats to the skillet and simmer until reduced by half, about 10 minutes. Add the honey and sherry vinegar and continue cooking until thick and syrupy.

5. Remove the game hens from the oven and pour the orange sauce over them. Continue roasting until the birds are cooked through, another 10 to 15 minutes.

6. Place the game hens on individual serving plates, ladling accumulated juices and the sauce over them. Garnish with the bacon pieces.

Tip: To prepare the kumquats, wash them, pat dry with paper towels, and slice horizontally into paper-thin slices, removing the seeds.

Nutrition Facts: 667 Calories | Fat 41g | Protein 57g | Carbohydrates 18g | Fiber 3g

Chicken Pad Thai

This recipe has all of the scrumptious flavors of the Thai restaurant staple—pungent fish sauce, tangy lime juice, seared chicken, fried eggs, and plenty of crunchy vegetables.

Serves: 4   *Prep time:* 10 minutes   *Cook time:* 15 minutes

2 tablespoons coconut oil, divided

4 eggs, whisked

1 pound chicken breast tenders

4 carrots, made into noodles with a spiralizer

1 tablespoon minced ginger

1 tablespoon minced garlic

3 tablespoons fish sauce

¼ cup lime juice

1 tablespoon honey

4 scallions, thinly sliced

½ cup minced fresh cilantro

½ cup roasted cashews

sea salt, to taste

freshly ground pepper, to taste

1. Heat a large skillet over medium-high heat. When it is very hot, add 1 tablespoon of the coconut oil. Tilt to coat the pan.

2. Pour the eggs into the pan. They will begin to cook immediately. Season with salt. When the eggs are mostly set, about 2 minutes, use a spatula to flip the omelet. It may break apart a little, and that's okay. Fry on the other side for 30 seconds. Fold into quarters and transfer to a cutting board. Slice into thin ribbons when cool enough to handle.

3. Return the skillet to the heat. Pat the chicken tenders dry with a paper towel. Season generously with salt and pepper. Sear until cooked through, about 5 minutes. Transfer to the cutting board.

4. Return the skillet to the heat. Add the remaining tablespoon of oil and cook the carrots for 3 minutes. They will still be crunchy. Add the ginger and garlic to the pan and cook for another 2 minutes, until very fragrant.

5. Whisk the fish sauce, lime juice, and honey in a small bowl and pour into the pan. Add the scallions and cook for 2 to 3 minutes.

6. Return the eggs and chicken to the pan and toss gently to mix everything. Transfer the pad thai to individual serving plates and garnish with the cilantro and cashews.

Tip: Cashews are a gray area. Technically, they're neither a tree nut nor a legume, even though they split like some legumes. Ultimately, listen to your body and eat what makes you feel good. Don't get too hung up on the botanical definition.

Nutrition Facts: 398 Calories | Fat 23g | Protein 36g | Carbohydrates 13g | Fiber 1g

Chicken Cassoulet

When you first embark on a lectin-avoidance diet, it might seem like your life will be filled with nothing but chicken over lettuce. With savory sausage, fresh vegetables, and bone-in chicken, this warming French stew proves that this diet is anything but boring! Enjoy with a dry sauvignon blanc or pinot noir.

Serves: 4   *Prep time:* 10 minutes   *Cook time:* 1 hour

Egg-Free, Nut-Free, Allergen-Free

4 ounces salt pork, cut into 1-inch pieces

4 bone-in, skin-on chicken thighs

4 bone-in, skin-on chicken drumsticks

2 garlic sausage links, casings removed and crumbled

1 small yellow onion, minced

2 carrots, minced

2 celery stalks, minced

1 tablespoon minced garlic

2 bay leaves

1 tablespoon fresh thyme leaves

4 cups Chicken Broth (page 171)

¼ cup dry white wine

sea salt, to taste

freshly ground pepper, to taste

1. Preheat the oven to 425°F.

2. Heat a cast-iron skillet over medium heat. Cook the salt pork until it renders most of its fat, about 10 minutes. Transfer the cooked pork to a separate dish.

3. Increase the heat to medium-high. Pat the chicken thighs and drumsticks dry with paper towels and season liberally with salt and pepper. Sear for 5 minutes on each side, or until gently browned. They will not be cooked through yet. Transfer to a separate dish.

4. Add the sausage to the pan and cook until just cooked through, about 4 minutes. Transfer to a separate dish.

5. Add the onion, carrots, celery, garlic, bay leaves, and thyme to the pan. Cook for 5 to 7 minutes, until nearly tender.

6. Add the chicken broth and white wine to the pan and bring to a simmer. Add the salt pork, chicken, and sausage to the pan. Transfer the pan to the oven and bake for 30 minutes, until the meat is browned and the stew is bubbling.

Tip: Make sure to read the label on the garlic sausage to ensure it does not contain nightshades.

Nutrition Facts: 504 Calories | Fat 33g | Protein 43g | Carbohydrates 5g | Fiber 1g

Duck Breast with Cabernet Thyme Reduction

Don't be intimidated by duck breast. The preparation requires a bit of precision, but it's really not difficult at all. Simply score the skin, making sure not to cut through to the meat, and then give it a good sear to render the delicious duck fat before transferring to the oven to finish. Seriously good eats! Pair it with Creamy Celeriac Puree (page 58) and Roasted Brussels Sprouts (page 67).

Serves: 4   *Prep time:* 5 minutes   *Cook time:* 22 minutes

Egg-Free, Nut-Free, Allergen-Free

4 (6-ounce) Muscovy duck breasts

1 shallot, halved

1 fresh thyme sprig

1 cup Cabernet or another full-bodied red wine

sea salt, to taste

freshly ground pepper, to taste

1. Preheat the oven to 350°F.

2. Heat a cast-iron skillet or another oven-proof skillet over medium-high heat until it is very hot.

3. Meanwhile, place the duck breasts on a cutting board and cut through the skin at 1-inch intervals in both directions, to yield a diamond pattern. Be careful not to cut all the way through to the meat. Season the duck liberally with salt and pepper.

4. Place the duck skin-side down into the pan and cook for 5 minutes, until the duck has rendered some of its fat. Flip and cook on the second side for 2 minutes.

5. Add the shallot and thyme to the pan and transfer to the oven. Roast for another 5 minutes.

6. Remove the duck to a cutting board to rest.

7. Carefully add the Cabernet to the pan and simmer over medium heat until reduced to about ⅓ of a cup, about 10 minutes. Discard the thyme and shallot.

8. Slice the duck on a bias and arrange on serving plates. Drizzle each portion with 1½ tablespoons of the wine reduction.

Nutrition Facts: 418 Calories | Fat 19g | Protein 46g | Carbohydrates 2g | Fiber 0g

Roasted Chicken Thighs with Kabocha, Parsnips, and Onion

Kabocha is my favorite squash because the texture is thick and meaty, and it caramelizes beautifully when roasted, transforming it almost into candy. Here it is roasted with carrots, parsnips, and red onion and paired with bone-in chicken thighs for a filling supper.

Serves: 4   *Prep time:* 10 minutes   *Cook time:* 50 to 55 minutes

Egg-Free, Nut-Free, Allergen-Free

1 small kabocha squash, halved vertically and sliced into ½-inch-thick half circles

2 large parsnips, halved lengthwise

6 carrots, halved lengthwise

1 red onion, cut into 8 wedges

4 tablespoons melted coconut oil, divided

4 bone-in, skin-on chicken thighs

sea salt, to taste

freshly ground pepper, to taste

1. Preheat the oven to 400°F.

2. Spread the squash, parsnips, carrots, and onion onto a rimmed baking sheet. Drizzle with 3 tablespoons of the coconut oil and toss the vegetables gently to coat. Season generously with salt and pepper. Transfer the pan to the oven and roast for 25 minutes.

4. Meanwhile, heat a large skillet over medium-high heat. Pat the chicken thighs dry with paper towels and season generously with salt and pepper. Add the remaining tablespoon of coconut oil to the pan and tilt to coat.

5. Sear the chicken thighs for 10 minutes, then flip and cook for another 5 minutes. Carefully remove the roasting vegetables from the oven and add the chicken to the baking sheet.

6. Continue roasting for another 15 to 20 minutes, or until the vegetables are deeply browned and the chicken is cooked through.

Nutrition Facts: 345 Calories | Fat 17g | Protein 17g | Carbohydrates 34g | Fiber 7g

---

Roasted Chicken Thighs with Mushrooms and Asparagus:
Prepare the recipe as directed above, but replace the squash, parsnips, carrots, and onion with 1 pint mushrooms, halved, 1 bunch asparagus, trimmed, and 1 tablespoon minced garlic. Toss the mushrooms, asparagus, and garlic with the coconut oil. Season with salt and pepper. Do not pre-roast the vegetables. Add them to the pan and roast for 15 to 20 minutes total, along with the chicken.

Nutrition Facts: 241 Calories | Fat 17g | Protein 17g | Carbohydrates 5g | Fiber 2g

---

CHAPTER SEVEN

BEEF, PORK, AND LAMB

Sesame Ginger Pork Lettuce Cups

These savory lettuce cups make a delicious appetizer or light lunch. Serve them with Peppercorn Beef and Broccoli Stir Fry (page 127) for a complete meal.

Serves: 4   *Prep time:* 10 minutes   *Cook time:* 7 minutes

Egg-Free

1 tablespoon toasted sesame oil

1 pound ground pork

1 tablespoon minced ginger

1 tablespoon minced garlic

2 tablespoons gluten-free soy sauce or coconut aminos

1 tablespoon lime juice

8 butter lettuce leaves

½ cup minced fresh cilantro

2 green onions, thinly sliced

1 carrot, julienned

¼ cup roughly chopped cashews

sea salt, to taste

freshly ground pepper, to taste

1. Heat the sesame oil in a large skillet over medium-high heat. Add the ground pork and cook for 5 minutes. Season with salt and pepper.

2. Add the ginger and garlic and continue cooking for 2 minutes. Add the soy sauce and lime juice, and cook for another minute until some of the liquid has evaporated.

3. Divide the pork between lettuce leaves and top with cilantro, green onions, carrot, and chopped cashews.

Tip: To cut the carrot, slice it into 2-inch pieces. Slice each piece into as thin a strip as you can. Stack a few strips on top of one another and cut into thin matchsticks.

Nutrition Facts: 431 Calories | Fat 31g | Protein 31g | Carbohydrates 6g | Fiber 1g

Slow-Cooker Beef and Vegetable Stew

Being on a special diet doesn't have to be stressful, especially when you can prepare a full dinner in just minutes in the morning and come home to a hearty beef and vegetable stew. If you have extra prep time, sear the beef in a skillet with a tablespoon of oil over high heat until browned on all sides before placing it into the slow cooker. This adds flavor, but it isn't essential, especially if you're using a good-quality grass-fed beef.

Serves: 4   *Prep time:* 10 minutes   *Cook time:* 8 hours

Egg-Free, Nut-Free, Allergen-Free

1 tablespoon extra-virgin olive oil	1 turnip, peeled and quartered
1 cup diced onions	2 parsnips, cut into 2-inch pieces
1 cup diced celery	1 cup white wine
2 cloves garlic, smashed	2 cups beef broth
1 bay leaf	sea salt, to taste
2 pounds beef chuck, cut into 1-inch pieces	freshly ground black pepper, to taste
2 carrots, cut into 2-inch pieces	

1. Coat the interior of a slow cooker with oil.

2. Layer the onion, celery, garlic, and bay leaf in the slow cooker.

3. Season the beef chuck generously with salt and pepper and set it atop the vegetables. Top with the carrots, turnip, and parsnips.

4. Pour in the wine and broth.

5. Cover and cook on low for 8 hours.

6. To serve, remove the beef and root vegetables, carrots, turnip, and parsnips to a serving bowl.

7. Use an immersion blender to puree the remaining vegetables and liquid. Adjust the seasoning and pour over the beef and vegetables.

Nutrition Facts: 444 Calories | Fat 18g | Protein 46g | Carbohydrates 23g | Fiber 6g

Chili Con Carne

I know what you're thinking—chili, how is that even possible without nightshades? While this version doesn't taste exactly like the original, it is pretty darn good, and thanks to beets and carrots, it looks similar, too.

Serves: 4 *Prep time:* 10 minutes *Cook time:* 1 hour 20 minutes

Egg-Free, Nut-Free, Allergen-Free

1 tablespoon extra-virgin olive oil

2 pounds beef chuck, cut into 1-inch pieces

1 cup diced onions

1 cup diced celery

1 cup diced carrots

1 cup peeled diced beets

2 cloves garlic, smashed

1 tablespoon ground cumin

1 teaspoon ground coriander

pinch cinnamon

1 cup red wine

2 cups beef broth

¼ cup minced cilantro, to serve

1 avocado, sliced, to serve

sea salt, to taste

freshly ground black pepper, to taste

1. Heat the oil in a large pot over high heat. Pat the beef dry with paper towels and season generously with salt and pepper. Sear the beef in the oil until well browned on all sides, about 10 minutes. Remove to a separate dish.

2. Add the onions, celery, carrots, and beets to the pot and cook for 5 minutes. Add the garlic to the pot and cook for another 2 minutes.

3. Add the cumin, coriander, and cinnamon. Cook for another minute to toast the spices.

4. Add the red wine and bring to a simmer for 2 minutes to cook off some of the alcohol.

5. Return the beef and any accumulated juices to the pan along with the beef broth.

6. Cover and cook over medium-low heat until the beef is very tender, about 1 hour.

7. Place the chili into serving bowls and garnish with cilantro and avocado.

Nutrition Facts: 470 Calories | Fat 25g | Protein 46g | Carbohydrates 16g | Fiber 6g

---

Carne Asada Burrito Bowl

This is one of my favorite lunchtime salads.

Serves: 4 *Prep time:* 5 minutes, plus at least 30 minutes to marinate *Cook time:* 6 to 10 minutes

Egg-Free, Nut-Free, Allergen-Free

2 tablespoons lime juice

2 tablespoons extra-virgin olive oil

1 teaspoon minced garlic

1 teaspoon ground cumin

1 teaspoon minced fresh oregano

1 teaspoon smoked black pepper

¼ teaspoon sea salt

1 (16-ounce) flank steak

4 cups shredded romaine lettuce

1 recipe Essential Roasted Sweet Potatoes (page 65)

½ cup Guacamole (page 164)

¼ cup minced red onion

¼ cup minced cilantro

1. Combine the lime juice, olive oil, garlic, cumin, oregano, pepper, and salt in a zip-top plastic bag. Add the flank steak and turn to coat. Allow to marinate for at least 30 minutes or up to 12 hours.

2. Heat a grill pan over medium-high heat. Sear the steak for 3 to 5 minutes on each side, until gently browned. Transfer to a cutting board to rest.

3. Divide the romaine lettuce between serving bowls. Top each bowl with ¼ of the roasted sweet potatoes.

4. Slice the steak into thin strips and divide between the salad bowls. Top each with 2 tablespoons of guacamole and garnish with red onion and cilantro.

Nutrition Facts: 477 Calories | Fat 30g | Protein 27g | Carbohydrates 29g | Fiber 7g

Peppercorn Beef and Broccoli Stir Fry

It's difficult, if not impossible, to navigate a Chinese restaurant menu and avoid nightshades. This version gets its heat from peppercorns and is complemented by a generous dose of ginger and garlic.

Serves: 2   *Prep time:* 5 minutes   *Cook time:* 18 minutes

Egg-Free, Nut-Free, Allergen-Free

1 tablespoon toasted coconut oil

1 (1-pound) boneless ribeye steak

1 tablespoon freshly ground pepper

1 tablespoon toasted sesame oil

1 head broccoli, cut into florets

1 tablespoon minced garlic

1 teaspoon minced ginger

¼ cup gluten-free soy sauce or coconut aminos

2 tablespoons lime juice

2 scallions, thinly sliced

sea salt, to taste

1. Heat a large skillet over medium-high heat. When it is hot, add the coconut oil to the pan. Pat the steak dry with paper towels. Season with salt and pepper. Sear for 5 minutes on each side for medium rare. Transfer to a cutting board to rest.

2. Return the pan to the heat and add the sesame oil. Sauté the broccoli until crisp-tender, about 5 to 7 minutes. Add the garlic and ginger to the pan and cook for 1 minute, reducing the heat if the garlic begins to burn. Add the soy sauce and lime juice and cook for 1 minute. Remove the pan from the heat.

3. Slice the steak in very thin slices and return it to the pan, along with any accumulated juices and the scallions. Give everything a good toss before serving.

Nutrition Facts: 314 Calories | Fat 25g | Protein 19g | Carbohydrates 4g | Fiber 1g

Sage Roasted Pork Tenderloin with Apricot Riesling Sauce

Sometimes the best recipes are the simplest, and that is certainly true of this quick and easy pan-roasted pork tenderloin. The apricot sauce is easy to pull together and complements the pungent sage and hearty pork tenderloin.

Serves: 4   *Prep time:* 5 minutes   *Cook time:* 25 to 30 minutes

Egg-Free, Nut-Free, Allergen-Free

2 cloves garlic

2 tablespoons minced fresh sage

½ teaspoon sea salt, plus more to taste

¼ teaspoon freshly ground pepper

2 tablespoons extra-virgin olive oil

1¼ pounds pork tenderloin

½ cup roughly chopped dried apricots

1 shallot, minced

1 cup Riesling

½ cup Chicken Broth (page 171)

1. Preheat the oven to 400°F.

2. Bash the garlic, sage, ½ teaspoon salt, and pepper in a mortar and pestle until it forms a paste. Whisk in the olive oil.

3. Pat the pork tenderloin dry with paper towels and rub the garlic and sage mixture over it.

4. Place the pork in a baking dish and roast for 25 to 30 minutes, or until cooked through and beginning to brown.

5. Meanwhile, combine the apricots, shallot, Riesling, and chicken broth in a small saucepan and bring to a simmer. Cook until the apricots are tender and the sauce has reduced to about ¾ cup. Use an immersion blender to puree until smooth. Season with salt.

6. Remove the pork from the oven and allow to rest for 10 minutes before slicing into medallions. Pour the apricot Riesling sauce over each portion.

Nutrition Facts: 390 Calories | Fat 19g | Protein 43g | Carbohydrates 11g | Fiber 1g

Rosemary Roasted Pork Tenderloin with Plum Wine Sauce:
Replace the sage with minced rosemary. Use dried plums and a full-bodied red wine in place of the Riesling.

Nutrition Facts: 390 Calories | Fat 19g | Protein 43g | Carbohydrates 11g | Fiber 1g

Grilled Coconut Ginger Pork Skewers

These grilled pork skewers are perfect for summer cookouts. They're even tasty at room temperature or chilled, so there's no rush to get dinner on the table. Serve with the pineapple salsa in the Grilled Mahi Mahi with Pineapple Salsa recipe (page 88).

Serves: 4   *Prep time:* 5 minutes, plus 30 minutes to marinate   *Cook time:* 8 to 10 minutes

Egg-Free, Nut-Free, Allergen-Free

½ cup coconut milk

2 tablespoons lime juice

1 tablespoon minced fresh ginger

1 tablespoon brown sugar

1 teaspoon ground turmeric

1 teaspoon ground coriander

½ teaspoon ground cumin

½ teaspoon sea salt

½ teaspoon freshly ground pepper

1¼ pounds pork tenderloin, cut into 1-inch pieces

1. Whisk the coconut milk, lime juice, ginger, brown sugar, turmeric, coriander, cumin, salt, and pepper together.

2. Pour the mixture over the pork and toss to coat. Allow the pork to marinate for 30 minutes while you preheat the grill, or up to 8 hours.

3. Thread the pork onto bamboo skewers, shaking off any excess marinade.

4. Grill over medium-high heat for 4 to 5 minutes on each side, or until cooked through and gently browned.

Nutrition Facts: 352 Calories | Fat 17g | Protein 42g | Carbohydrates 6g | Fiber 0g

Mojo Pork Tenderloin

Freshly squeezed orange and lime juices, ground cumin, and fresh cilantro infuse pork tenderloin with flavor in this classic Cuban recipe. Enjoy with Mashed Plantains with Bacon and Fennel (page 62) for a taste of the Caribbean.

Serves: 4   *Prep time:* 10 minutes, plus 8 hours to marinate   *Cook time:* 25 minutes

Egg-Free, Nut-Free, Allergen-Free

¼ cup extra-virgin olive oil

½ cup minced fresh cilantro

4 cloves garlic, minced

¼ cup freshly squeezed orange juice

3 tablespoons freshly squeezed lime juice

1 tablespoon minced fresh oregano

1 teaspoon ground cumin

1 teaspoon sea salt

½ teaspoon freshly ground pepper

1¼ pounds pork tenderloin

1. Combine the olive oil, cilantro, garlic, orange juice, lime juice, oregano, cumin, salt, and pepper in a large zip-top plastic bag. Add the pork tenderloin. Squeeze all of the excess air from the bag and seal it. Marinate in the refrigerator for 8 hours.

2. Remove the pork tenderloin from the marinade, shaking off any excess.

3. Preheat the oven to 325°F.

4. Heat a large oven-proof skillet over medium-high heat. When it is hot, add the pork tenderloin. Sear on all sides until gently browned, about 10 minutes total.

5. Transfer the pork to the oven and continue cooking for another 15 minutes, or until the pork is cooked through. Allow to rest for 10 minutes before slicing into medallions.

Nutrition Facts: 416 Calories | Fat 25g | Protein 42g | Carbohydrates 2g | Fiber <1g

Peppercorn-Crusted Pork Chops with Endive

Instead of coating cuts of meat with flour, I like to give them a nice crust of peppercorns and sea salt. The peppercorns infuse the pork chops with flavor as they rest after cooking. Be careful not to overcook!

Serves: 4   *Prep time:* 5 minutes   *Cook time:* 24 to 26 minutes

Egg-Free, Nut-Free, Allergen-Free

4 tablespoons olive oil, divided

4 (6-ounce) bone-in pork chops

2 tablespoons coarsely ground peppercorns

1 teaspoon sea salt

2 heads endive, halved lengthwise

1 teaspoon minced garlic

1 lemon, zest and juice

½ cup Chicken Broth (page 171)

sea salt, to taste

1. Heat a large skillet over medium-high heat until very hot. Add 2 tablespoons of the olive oil and heat until hot but not smoking.

2. Pat the pork chops dry with paper towels and season with the coarsely ground peppercorns and sea salt. Sear on each side for 6 to 8 minutes, until cooked through. Remove to a separate dish and cover to keep warm.

3. Add the remaining 2 tablespoons of olive oil to the pan. When it is hot, add the endives, cut-sides down. Get a good sear on the first side until well browned, about 5 minutes. Turn over and add the garlic, lemon zest and juice, and chicken broth to the pan. Cover and cook for 5 minutes, until the endives are soft. Serve alongside the pork chops.

Nutrition Facts: 380 Calories | Fat 24g | Protein 35g | Carbohydrates 10g | Fiber 10g

Pan-Seared Pork Chops with Browned Mushrooms

Sweet Marsala wine, savory browned mushrooms, and fresh herbs are the perfect complement to pan-seared pork chops.

Serves: 4   *Prep time:* 5 minutes   *Cook time:* 22 minutes

Egg-Free, Nut-Free, Allergen-Free

2 tablespoons extra-virgin olive oil, divided

4 (8-ounce) boneless, center-cut pork chops

2 cups sliced crimini mushrooms

1 tablespoons minced shallots

2 large cloves garlic, minced

1 teaspoon minced fresh thyme

½ teaspoon minced fresh rosemary

¼ cup Marsala

sea salt, to taste

freshly ground pepper, to taste

1. Heat a large skillet over medium-high heat. When it is very hot, add 1 tablespoon of the oil.

2. Pat the pork chops dry with paper towels and season generously with salt and pepper. Sear the pork chops for 5 minutes on each side. Transfer to a cutting board to rest.

3. Add the remaining tablespoon of oil to the pan. When it is hot, add the mushrooms. Cook until well browned on each side, about 7 minutes total. You may need to do this in batches to prevent the mushrooms from crowding the pan.

4. Add the shallots, garlic, thyme, and rosemary to the pan and cook until fragrant and the shallots begin to soften, about 3 minutes. Add the Marsala to the pan and cook until it is mostly evaporated, about 2 minutes.

5. Top each pork chop with a generous scoop of the cooked mushrooms.

Nutrition Facts: 333 Calories | Fat 16g | Protein 47g | Carbohydrates 4g | Fiber <1g

Costa Rican Coffee-Glazed Ribeye Steak

I made this recipe while on a surf trip in Encinitas, California. We had a massive steak to grill and a limited pantry in the vacation rental. But, with rum leftover from the night before, plenty of strong coffee, and a few spices, I pulled this together. It was surprisingly flavorful and made the grilled steak unforgettable.

Serves: 2 to 4   *Prep time:* 10 minutes   *Cook time:* 40 minutes

Egg-Free, Nut-Free, Allergen-Free

1 cup strong coffee	1 shallot, halved
½ cup dark rum	¼ cup red wine vinegar
1 teaspoon peppercorns	¼ cup brown sugar
1 teaspoon coriander seeds	1 pound boneless ribeye steak

1. Preheat a grill or grill pan to medium-high heat.

2. Bring the coffee, rum, peppercorns, coriander, shallot, red wine vinegar, and sugar to a simmer in a small saucepan. Cook for 20 minutes, until reduced to about ¾ cup. Strain, discarding the shallot and spices, and allow to cool.

3. Pour half of the glaze over the ribeye steak, turning to coat.

4. Brush the grill grates with oil using a paper towel. Grill the steak on one side for 10 minutes until you get a good sear. Flip the steak and brush with additional marinade. Grill for another 10 minutes, brushing with the glaze occasionally.

5. Allow to rest for 10 minutes before slicing and serving.

Tip: If you have the time, allow the ribeye to sit in the marinade overnight in the refrigerator.

Nutrition Facts: 439 Calories | Fat 34g | Protein 34g | Carbohydrates 12g | Fiber 0g

Short-Rib Ragu Fettuccine

There are few meals more luxurious than slow-roasted beef short ribs atop fresh fettuccine.

Serves: 4   *Prep time:* 10 minutes   *Cook time:* 2 hours 15 minutes

1 pound beef short ribs

2 celery stalks, diced

2 carrots, diced

1 red onion, diced

1 teaspoon minced fresh thyme

1 teaspoon minced fresh rosemary

1 cup red wine

2 tablespoons gluten-free soy sauce or coconut aminos

1 recipe Grain-Free Fettuccine (page 180) or Cappello's gluten-free fettuccine

sea salt, to taste

freshly ground pepper, to taste

1. Heat a large cast-iron skillet over medium-high heat. Season the short ribs liberally with salt and pepper. Place them meat-side down into the skillet and sear until well browned, about 10 minutes.

2. Flip the short ribs and add the celery, carrots, onion, thyme, and rosemary to the pan. Saute for 5 minutes, until the vegetables begin to soften.

3. Pour in the red wine and soy sauce. Cover the pan tightly with foil or an oven-proof lid. Bake for 2 hours.

4. Remove the beef bones from the beef and shred the meat with a fork. Return the meat to the pan. Adjust the seasoning, as needed.

5. Bring a large pot of salted water to a boil. Cook the pasta for 90 seconds, drain, and divide between serving dishes.

6. Ladle the short-rib ragu over each portion of pasta.

Nutrition Facts: 692 Calories | Fat 40g | Protein 26g | Carbohydrates 32g | Fiber 5g

Beef Bourguignon

This classic French stew has all the elegance of meal at a fine dining restaurant. But, it uses easy-to-find ingredients and basic cooking techniques. The trick is to buy the best ingredients you can afford. I prefer grass-fed beef in this recipe. Make sure the wine is something you would want to drink. Serve with Creamy Celeriac Puree (page 58).

Serves: 4   *Prep time:* 10 minutes   *Cook time:* 2 hours

Egg-Free, Nut-Free, Allergen-Free

1 tablespoon extra-virgin olive oil

2 pounds beef chuck

2 cups cremini mushrooms, halved

2 cups blanched pearl onions

4 carrots, cut into 2-inch pieces

1 sprig fresh rosemary

1 sprig fresh thyme

2 cups dry red wine, such as pinot noir

2 cups beef broth

1 teaspoon sugar

sea salt, to taste

freshly ground pepper, to taste

1. Heat a large pot over medium-high heat. Add the olive oil.

2. Pat the beef dry with paper towels and season generously with salt and pepper. Sear the beef in the hot oil until well browned on all sides. This will take at least 10 minutes because you will have to do it in batches so as not to crowd the pan.

3. Remove the beef to a separate dish. It will not yet be cooked through.

4. Add the mushrooms to the pan and sear for 2 minutes until gently browned. Add the onions, carrots, rosemary, thyme, red wine, and beef broth. Bring to a simmer. Return the beef and any accumulated juices to the pan.

5. Cover and cook for 1 hour. Remove the lid from the pan and continue cooking for 45 minutes, allowing the liquid to reduce.

The meat should be tender enough that it slices easily with a fork. Stir in the sugar to round out the sauce.

Tip: The stew gets better as it sits. So, prepare it a day ahead of time and reheat it before serving.

Nutrition Facts: 513 Calories | Fat 16g | Protein 55g | Carbohydrates 3g | Fiber 3g

---

Zuppa Toscana

Creamy, savory zuppa Toscana—or Tuscan soup—is a cream-based soup with Italian sausage and potatoes. In this version, I use ground pork, crushed fennel seed, white sweet potatoes, and creamy coconut milk for a nightshade-free and dairy-free version.

Serves: 4   *Prep time:* 10 minutes   *Cook time:* 40 minutes

Egg-Free, Nut-Free, Allergen-Free

1 tablespoon extra-virgin olive oil

1 pound ground pork

1 teaspoon crushed fennel seed

2 tablespoons minced garlic

1 yellow onion, minced

2 large white sweet potatoes, peeled and cut into 1-inch pieces

4 cups Chicken Broth (page 171)

1 cup full-fat coconut milk

2 cup shredded kale

sea salt, to taste

freshly ground pepper, to taste

1. Heat the olive oil in a large pot over medium-high heat. Cook the pork and fennel seed until well browned, about 10 minutes. Use a slotted spoon to transfer the pork to a separate dish.

2. Add the garlic and onion to the pot and cook for 5 minutes until the onion begins to soften. Do not allow the garlic to burn.

3. Add the sweet potatoes, chicken broth, and coconut milk along with the cooked pork and any accumulated juices. Season with salt and pepper. Bring to a simmer and cook until the sweet potatoes are tender, about 20 minutes.

4. Add the kale to the pot and cook for 5 minutes, until it's just softened.

Nutrition Facts: 570 Calories | Fat 39g | Protein 34g | Carbohydrates 23g | Fiber 4g

Chimichurri Grilled Lamb Chops

I love the Argentine flavors in this easy grilled lamb recipe. The grassy flavors of the parsley and mint complement the gaminess of the lamb, while pungent garlic and red wine vinegar amp up the flavor.

Serves: 4 *Prep time:* 5 minutes, plus at least 30 minutes to marinate *Cook time:* 16 to 20 minutes

Egg-Free, Nut-Free, Allergen-Free

4 cloves garlic, roughly chopped

½ red onion, roughly chopped

½ cup roughly chopped fresh parsley

¼ cup roughly chopped fresh mint

2 tablespoons red wine vinegar

¼ cup extra-virgin olive oil

½ teaspoon sea salt

½ teaspoon freshly ground pepper

4 (6- to 8-ounce) lamb shoulder chops

1. Place the garlic, onion, parsley, mint, red wine vinegar, olive oil, salt, and pepper into a blender. Puree until smooth. Spread this mixture over the lamb chops. Allow to marinate for at least 30 minutes or up to 8 hours in the refrigerator.

2. Preheat a grill to medium-high heat. Remove the lamb chops from the marinade, shaking off any excess. Grill the lamb chops for about 8 to 10 minutes on each side, until cooked through.

Nutrition Facts: 353 Calories | Fat 23g | Protein 35g | Carbohydrates 2g | Fiber 1g

Meatloaf

Traditional meatloaf is bound with bread crumbs and smothered in ketchup. This version uses almond flour and vegetables to hold things together and opts for a few strips of bacon on top instead. For familiar flavors, go with the Tomato-Free Marinara Sauce (page 168).

Serves: 8   *Prep time:* 15 minutes   *Cook time:* 1 hour 10 minutes

1 tablespoon extra-virgin olive oil

1 cup minced onion

½ cup minced celery

½ cup minced carrots

1 tablespoon minced garlic

1 teaspoon minced rosemary

¼ cup minced parsley

½ cup almond flour

1 egg, whisked

1 teaspoon sea salt

1 teaspoon freshly ground pepper

1 pound ground beef

1 pound ground pork

4 slices applewood-smoked bacon

1. Preheat the oven to 350°F.

2. Heat a large skillet over medium heat. When it is hot, add the oil. Cook the onion, celery, carrots, garlic, rosemary, and parsley for 8 to 10 minutes, until soft.

3. In a large mixing bowl, mix the almond flour, egg, salt, and pepper until they form a thick paste. Add the cooked vegetables, beef, and pork. Use your hands to combine everything, being careful not to overmix.

4. Transfer the meat to a loaf pan and top with the bacon slices. Bake for 1 hour or until the meatloaf is cooked through.

5. Slice into 8 thick slices and serve.

Nutrition Facts: 434 Calories | Fat 34g | Protein 28g | Carbohydrates 4g | Fiber 2g

Meatballs and Marinara: Prepare the meatloaf ingredients as described above, omitting the bacon. Form the mixture into 16 balls. Heat the skillet used for cooking the onions and sear the meatballs on all sides until browned. Place them into a large baking dish. Pour 1 recipe Tomato-Free Marinara Sauce over them. Bake for 30 minutes.

Nutrition Facts: 482 Calories | Fat 40g | Protein 28g | Carbohydrates 15g | Fiber 4g

Rosemary Prime Rib Roast

My husband works at a church, and every year, the staff Christmas party happens at the pastor's house. The dish people most look forward to is his rosemary roasted prime rib roast. Some years, we're lucky enough to score a few slices to take home afterward! Now, you can enjoy the holiday favorite any time of the year.

Serves: 8   *Prep time:* 10 minutes, plus 8 hours resting time   *Cook time:* 1½ to 2 hours

Egg-Free, Nut-Free, Allergen-Free

2 tablespoons minced garlic

1 tablespoon minced rosemary

1 teaspoon sea salt

1 teaspoon freshly ground pepper

3 tablespoons olive oil

1 center-cut prime rib roast, 3 to 4 pounds

1. Mix the garlic, rosemary, sea salt, pepper, and olive oil in a mortar and pestle until it forms a thick paste. Coat the rib roast in this mixture and refrigerate for 8 hours or overnight.

2. Remove the meat from the refrigerator at least 1 hour before placing in the oven.

3. Preheat the oven to 450°F. Roast uncovered for 30 minutes to develop a nice crust on the exterior.

4. Reduce the heat to 325°F. Roast for another 1 to 1½ hours or until the roast reaches an internal temperature of 140°F. Remove to a cutting board and allow to rest for 20 minutes before slicing and serving.

Nutrition Facts: 413 Calories | Fat 25g | Protein 43g | Carbohydrates 0g | Fiber 0g

Mediterranean Lamb Kebabs

Ground sumac has an unmistakable tangy flavor that stands up well to the strong flavor of lamb. You can find it in well-stocked grocery stores, such as Whole Foods, or online.

Serves: 4   *Prep time:* 5 minutes   *Cook time:* 15 minutes

Egg-Free, Nut-Free, Allergen-Free

1 pound thick-cut boneless lamb chops, cut into 1-inch cubes

1 red onion, cut into ½-inch pieces

2 tablespoons olive oil

1 teaspoon ground cumin

1 teaspoon ground sumac (optional)

¼ cup tahini

1 tablespoon minced fresh garlic

2 tablespoons lemon juice

2 tablespoons red wine vinegar, divided

1 cucumber, peeled, seeded, and diced

1 cup Kalamata olives, pitted

sea salt, to taste

freshly ground pepper, to taste

1. Preheat the oven to 400°F.

2. Thread the lamb and onion onto bamboo skewers. Coat them thoroughly in the olive oil and season with salt, pepper, cumin, and sumac, if using.

3. Roast uncovered for 15 minutes, or until the meat is cooked to your desired level of doneness.

4. While the meat cooks, whisk together the tahini, garlic, lemon juice, and 1 tablespoon of the red wine vinegar.

5. Combine the diced cucumber and Kalamata olives, and toss with the remaining tablespoon of red wine vinegar. Serve the kebabs with the tahini sauce for dipping alongside the cucumber salad.

Nutrition Facts: 359 Calories | Fat 25g | Protein 27g | Carbohydrates 9g | Fiber 2g

CHAPTER EIGHT

DESSERTS

Coconut Dream Bars

If you wanted to enjoy these no-bake coconut chocolate pecan bars as a snack or even for breakfast, I wouldn't blame you. They're loaded with healthy fats and have a scant amount of sugar from the maple syrup.

Serves: 12   *Prep time:* 10 minutes   *Cook time:* none

Egg-Free, Vegan

3 tablespoons unsweetened cocoa powder

1¼ cups crushed pecans, divided

¼ teaspoon sea salt

2 dates, pitted and roughly chopped

½ cup coconut oil (in solid form)

1 vanilla bean, scraped

3 tablespoons maple syrup

1¼ cups shredded unsweetened coconut flakes

2 tablespoons cacao nibs (optional)

1. Combine the cocoa powder, 1 cup of the pecans, and sea salt in a food processor, and pulse until it resembles coarse sand. Add the dates and pulse until the mixture comes together.

2. Press mixture into the bottom of an 8 x 5-inch baking dish.

3. In a separate dish, combine the coconut oil, vanilla, and maple syrup. Stir in 1 cup of the shredded coconut. Spoon this mixture over the cocoa-pecan crust and smooth with a spatula or the back of a spoon.

4. Top with the remaining pecans, coconut flakes, and cacao nibs, if using. Cut into 12 portions and top with parchment paper.

5. Refrigerate for at least 15 minutes.

Tip: Make sure to let these bars chill properly before slicing, especially if you make them during warm weather.

Nutrition Facts: 240 Calories | Fat 24g | Protein 2g | Carbohydrates 9g | Fiber 3g

Bourbon Vanilla Chocolate Truffles

I have been making chocolate truffles for years, but these have to be the easiest and most delicious. They have a smooth, creamy texture with just the perfect hit of bourbon and vanilla. If the chocolate is too hard to roll into balls after refrigerating, allow it to sit out on the counter for about 15 minutes before rolling the truffles.

Yield: 24 small truffles (3 truffles per serving) *Prep time:* 15 minutes, plus 1 hour to chill *Cook time:* 5 minutes

Egg-Free, Nut-Free, Allergen-Free, Vegan

⅓ cup full-fat coconut milk

¼ teaspoon sea salt

7 ounces dark chocolate (70 to 80 percent cacao), finely chopped

1½ tablespoons bourbon vanilla extract

¼ cup unsweetened cocoa powder

1. Bring the coconut milk and sea salt to a gentle simmer in a small pot over low heat.

2. Add the chocolate pieces and heat until nearly melted, stirring occasionally, about 3 minutes.

3. Add the vanilla extract and stir until just combined.

4. Place the pot into the refrigerator and chill until mostly hard, about 1 hour.

5. Place the cocoa powder in a shallow bowl.

6. Use a teaspoon to scoop the chocolate into small balls. Roll them briefly in your hands to shape, but not too long, or they will melt.

7. Roll the balls in the cocoa powder, shaking off any excess, and then place on a serving tray.

8. Cover and refrigerate until ready to serve. Allow to sit at room temperature for 10 minutes before serving.

Nutrition Facts: 158 Calories | Fat 14g | Protein 3g | Carbohydrates 8g | Fiber 5g

Paleo Thin Mints

This recipe appeared in one of my earlier cookbooks, *Sheet Pan Paleo*, and was quickly deemed by readers worth the entire purchase price of the book. I hope you find them as delicious as we have!

Yield: 24 cookies   *Prep time:* 10 minutes   *Cook time:* none

Egg-Free, Vegan

1 cup Medjool dates

1 cup walnuts

3 tablespoons cocoa powder

¼ teaspoon peppermint oil

1 tablespoon cacao nibs

½ cup Magic Chocolate Sauce (page 150)

sea salt, to taste

1. Combine the dates and walnuts in a food processor and grind until fairly smooth. Add the cocoa powder and a pinch of sea salt and pulse until thoroughly integrated. Sprinkle in the peppermint oil and pulse several more times. Finally, add the cacao nibs and pulse once or twice more, just until integrated.

2. Line a sheet pan with parchment paper. Form the dough into small, flat cookie shapes and place them on the pan. Place the pan in the freezer for 20 minutes. You do not want to freeze the cookies, just thoroughly chill them. If you want to make the filling ahead of time, simply store the cookies in the refrigerator until ready to coat with the chocolate.

3. One at a time, dunk the cookies into the chocolate oil, shaking off any excess, and return to the sheet pan.

4. Place in the freezer for 5 minutes just to firm up again. Store cookies in the refrigerator.

Nutrition Facts: 100 Calories | Fat 8g | Protein 1g | Carbohydrates 8g | Fiber 2g

Frozen Chocolate Banana Chips

These sweet treats make the perfect after-school snack or dessert.

Serves: 12   *Prep time:* 5 minutes, plus 1 hour to chill   *Cook time:* none
Egg-Free, Nut-Free, Allergen-Free, Vegan

   4 bananas, sliced in ½-inch-thick pieces

   ½ cup Magic Chocolate Sauce (page 150)

1. Spread the sliced bananas out on a baking sheet lined with parchment paper. Freeze until solid, about 50 minutes.

2. Dip the banana slices in the chocolate sauce and return to the baking tray. Place in the freezer for 5 to 10 minutes to harden. Store in a covered container in the freezer.

Nutrition Facts: 122 Calories | Fat 10g | Protein 1g | Carbohydrates 11g | Fiber 2g

Magic Chocolate Sauce

What makes this sauce magical? It hardens on contact with chilled ingredients, making it perfect for drizzling over ice cream or dipping frozen treats in. Keep this chocolate sauce on hand and simply set out at room temperature or in a bowl of warm water to liquefy.

Yield: ½ cup   *Prep time:* 5 minutes   *Cook time:* none

Egg-Free, Nut-Free, Allergen-Free, Vegan

¼ cup cocoa powder	1 tablespoon maple syrup
½ cup coconut oil, melted	sea salt, to taste

Whisk together the cocoa powder, coconut oil, maple syrup, and a tiny pinch of sea salt in a shallow bowl. Store in a covered container in the refrigerator.

Nutrition Facts: 130 Calories | Fat 14g | Protein 1g | Carbohydrates 3g | Fiber 1g

Chocolate Almond Butter Cups

After years of eating a diet without much sugar, I have come to prefer these lightly sweetened treats over the sugary confections that proliferate around Halloween. You know which ones I'm talking about. Unlike the chocolate peanut butter cups, these have no dairy or refined sugar.

Serves: 12   *Prep time:* 10 minutes, plus 40 minutes resting time   *Cook time:* none

Egg-Free, Vegan

½ cup coconut oil, melted

1 cup creamy almond butter, divided

¼ cup maple syrup

½ cup unsweetened cocoa powder

½ teaspoon sea salt, divided

1. Pour the coconut oil, ½ cup of almond butter, and the maple syrup into a blender. Pulse to combine.

2. Add the cocoa powder and sea salt. Blend until thoroughly combined.

3. Divide about half of the mixture between 12 lined muffin cups. An easy way to do this is to use measuring spoons to dole out about 2 tablespoons per cup. Place in the refrigerator for about 10 minutes to firm slightly.

4. Divide the remaining almond butter between each of the chocolate cups. If you use a measuring spoon, it will be about 2 teaspoons. Sprinkle each with a small pinch of sea salt, then pour the remaining chocolate mixture over the top.

5. Refrigerate until set, about 30 more minutes. Store in the refrigerator in a covered container.

Tip: If you swap maple syrup for agave, use only 3 tablespoons of agave; it is 25 percent sweeter.

Nutrition Facts: 235 Calories | Fat 21g | Protein 4g | Carbohydrates 11g | Fiber 3g

Maple Tahini Ice Cream

The first time I tried this ice cream, I was blown away with how delicious it is and how much it tastes like a dairy-based peanut butter ice cream. The miso adds an umami quality to the ice cream and is made using gut-friendly fermented soy, but you can omit it for a soy-free version. It is especially delicious drizzled with Magic Chocolate Sauce (page 150).

Yield: 7 (½-cup) servings *Prep time:* 5 minutes, plus chill time *Cook time:* none

Egg-Free, Vegan

1 (15-ounce) can full-fat coconut milk

1 cup unsweetened Almond Milk (page 169)

⅓ cup tahini

½ cup maple syrup

1 tablespoon white miso

1 tablespoon vanilla extract

1. Combine all of the ingredients in a blender and puree until smooth, scraping down the sides as needed.

2. Pour the mixture into an ice cream maker and follow the manufacturer's instructions.

3. Transfer the ice cream to a covered container and freeze until firm. Allow to thaw on the countertop for 10 minutes before serving.

Tip: To make this nut free, swap the almond milk with 8 ounces of light coconut milk.

Nutrition Facts: 194 Calories | Fat 13g | Protein 3g | Carbohydrates 17g | Fiber 1g

German Chocolate Ice Cream

Coconut, almonds, and chocolate are a natural combination in German chocolate cake. This ice cream plays up that flavor pairing with coconut milk and almond milk. Sprinkle with toasted coconut and toasted almonds for a real treat.

Serves: 8   *Prep time:* minutes   *Cook time:* minutes

Egg-Free, Nut-Free, Allergen-Free, Vegan

1 cup unsweetened Almond Milk (page 169)

1 (14-ounce) can full-fat coconut milk

1 tablespoon brewed coffee

¼ teaspoon sea salt

2 tablespoons coconut palm sugar or brown sugar

4 ounces dairy-free dark chocolate (at least 75 percent cacao)

1. Heat the almond milk, coconut milk, coffee, sea salt, and palm sugar in a medium sauce pan. When the sugar is dissolved, add the dark chocolate and melt over very low heat until nearly melted. Remove from heat.

2. Cover the surface of the mixture with parchment paper or plastic wrap to prevent a skin from forming. Chill the mixture in the refrigerator until completely cooled.

3. Pour the mixture into the ice cream maker and allow to churn for about 20 minutes, or until thick and voluminous. Enjoy immediately or freeze until solid.

Nutrition Facts: 143 Calories | Fat 12g | Protein 2g | Carbohydrates 10g | Fiber 2g

Maple Chocolate Torte

This may be one of the best desserts I have ever made. It is complex and perfectly balanced with a salted hazelnut crust and a creamy maple and bourbon chocolate ganache filling. The crust has a similar texture to graham cracker crusts, and the filling is richly dense while remaining easily sliceable.

Serves: 12   *Prep time:* 10 minutes, plus 2 to 3 hours to cool   *Cook time:* 15 minutes

Egg-Free, Vegan

2 cups ground hazelnuts (about 200 grams)

1 tablespoon coconut palm sugar or brown sugar

1 teaspoon plus 1 pinch sea salt

2 tablespoons palm shortening or vegan butter, melted

3 teaspoons vanilla extract, divided

¾ cup coconut cream, divided

½ cup maple syrup

3 tablespoons bourbon (optional)

6 ounces 100% cacao chocolate, such as Guittard, roughly chopped

1. Preheat the oven to 350°F.

2. In a small mixing bowl, combine the hazelnuts, sugar, and teaspoon of sea salt. Drizzle in the melted butter or shortening and 1 teaspoon of the vanilla extract. Stir to mix thoroughly.

3. Press the mixture into a 9-inch tart pan with removable bottom.

4. Place the tart pan on a larger baking sheet and bake for 10 minutes. Cool on a cooling rack.

5. To make the filling, bring ½ cup of the coconut cream, maple syrup, remaining vanilla extract, remaining sea salt, and bourbon, if using, to a simmer in a small saucepan. Remove from the heat.

6. Stir in the chocolate with a spatula and then allow to rest for 5 minutes. Stir again until the chocolate is melted.

7. Stir in the remaining ¼ cup of coconut cream to cool the mixture.

8. Pour into the prepared tart shell and refrigerate until set, 2 to 3 hours.

Nutrition Facts: 273 Calories | Fat 23g | Protein 5g | Carbohydrates 17g | Fiber 4g

Chinese Five-Spice Pear Crisp

I was out of ground ginger and decided to use Chinese five spice powder in place of the usual spices. The cardamom and black pepper were surprisingly awesome additions to the sweet dessert. Pears break down quickly when baked, making them perfect in a crisp because the topping also cooks quickly.

Serves: 8   *Prep time:* 10 minutes   *Cook time:* 25 minutes

Egg-Free, Vegan

½ cup palm shortening, plus more for coating the pan

8 pears, peeled, cored, and diced

¼ cup tapioca starch, divided

1 tablespoon plus 1 teaspoon Chinese five-spice powder

1 cup blanched almond flour

¼ teaspoon sea salt

¼ cup brown sugar

1. Preheat the oven to 350°F. Coat the interior of an 8 x 8-inch baking dish with palm shortening.

2. Place the pears into the baking dish and season with 2 tablespoons of the tapioca starch and 1 teaspoon of the five-spice powder.

3. Mix the remaining 2 tablespoons tapioca starch, 1 tablespoon five-spice powder, almond flour, sea salt, and brown sugar in a bowl. Add the palm shortening and use a fork to mix it until it crumbles easily between your fingers.

4. Sprinkle the crumbly topping over the pears. Bake for 25 minutes until the top is gently browned and the filling is bubbling.

Nutrition Facts: 245 Calories | Fat 14g | Protein 4g | Carbohydrates 33g | Fiber 6g

Black and Blueberry Crisp: Replace the pears with 2 cups of fresh blackberries and 3 cups of fresh blueberries. Omit the five-spice powder and add 1 teaspoon grated lemon zest to the filling.

Nutrition Facts: 214 Calories | Fat 14g | Protein 4g | Carbohydrates 25g | Fiber 5g

Vanilla Peach Crumble: Replace the pears with 8 fresh peaches. Omit the five-spice powder and add ¼ teaspoon freshly ground nutmeg and 1 tablespoon vanilla extract to the filling.

Nutrition Facts: 207 Calories | Fat 14g | Protein 4g | Carbohydrates 23g | Fiber 4g

Roasted Apples with Thyme and Red Wine

Fruit makes an easy and elegant dessert, especially when you infuse it with unlikely herbs. Earthy thyme, sweet maple syrup, and robust red wine blend to complement the roasted apples and form a thick, sweet syrup.

Serves: 4   *Prep time:* 5 minutes   *Cook time:* 40 minutes

Egg-Free, Nut-Free, Allergen-Free, Vegan

2 tablespoons coconut oil, divided

2 apples, peeled, halved, and cored

1 tablespoon minced fresh thyme leaves

pinch sea salt

1 teaspoon ground cinnamon

½ cup red wine

¼ cup maple syrup

1. Preheat the oven to 400°F. Coat the interior of an 8 x 8-inch baking dish with 1 tablespoon of the coconut oil.

2. Place the apples cut-side down into the baking dish, rub them with the second tablespoon of coconut oil, and sprinkle with the fresh thyme and a pinch of sea salt.

3. Bake for 20 minutes.

4. Add the wine and maple syrup to dish, turning the apples to let the liquid go underneath them, and continue baking for another 20 minutes, or until the apples are very tender and the wine has reduced to a thick, syrupy sauce.

Nutrition Facts: 172 Calories | Fat 7g | Protein <1g | Carbohydrates 24g | Fiber 2g

Rosemary Roasted Pears: For a healthier version without alcohol and less sugar, swap the apples for pears, use rosemary in place of the thyme, omit the wine, and reduce the maple syrup to 2 tablespoons. Add the maple syrup during the final 10 minutes of baking, after roasting the pears for 30 minutes.

Nutrition Facts: 120 Calories | Fat 7g | Protein <1g | Carbohydrates 16g | Fiber 2g

Baked Peaches with Macadamia Mousse

This recipe works well even if your peaches aren't soft and juicy—actually, it works even better if the peaches are on the firm side.

Serves: 4   *Prep time:* 5 minutes   *Cook time:* 20 minutes

Egg-Free, Vegan

2 peaches, halved

½ cup Sweet Vanilla Macadamia Mousse (page 170)

1 teaspoon ground cinnamon

1. Preheat the oven to 400°F.

2. Place the peaches into an 8 x 10-inch baking dish cut-side up. Scoop 2 tablespoons of the macadamia mousse into the center of each peach. Sprinkle with cinnamon.

3. Bake for 20 minutes.

Tip: This recipe also works with nectarines.

Nutrition Facts: 155 Calories | Fat 13g | Protein 1g | Carbohydrates 11g | Fiber 2g

CHAPTER NINE

SAUCES, CONDIMENTS, AND OTHER BASICS

Garlic Aioli

Serve this tangy aioli with Crab Cakes (page 75) or Root Vegetable Latkes (page 35), or enjoy as a dip for Essential Roasted Sweet Potatoes cut into spears (page 65). The key to creating an emulsified sauce—instead of an oily mess—is to very slowly integrate the oil. Too quickly won't work. Be patient and go slowly.

Yield: 8 (1-tablespoon) servings   *Prep time:* 5 minutes   *Cook time:* none
Nut-Free, Vegetarian

1 egg yolk

1 teaspoon lemon juice

1 small clove garlic, minced

2 tablespoons extra-virgin olive oil

⅓ cup canola oil

1. Combine the egg yolk, lemon juice, and garlic in a small, slightly warmed bowl.

2. Drizzle in the olive oil a few drops at a time, whisking constantly. Drizzle in the canola oil in the same manner, to emulsify the oil.

3. Store in a covered container in the refrigerator for up to 3 days.

Nutrition Facts: 116 Calories | Fat 13g | Protein 0g | Carbohydrates 0g | Fiber 0g

Pesto

Most prepared pesto contains cheese, so I make my own. This version, like most traditional pesto, contains pine nuts. But, you can make it without nuts if you prefer.

Yield: 8 (2-tablespoon) servings   *Prep time:* 5 minutes   *Cook time:* none
Egg-Free, Vegan

2 cups loosely packed fresh basil	¼ cup extra-virgin olive oil
2 cloves garlic, minced	¼ cup finely ground, toasted pine nuts
2 teaspoons lemon juice	

1. Place the basil, garlic, lemon juice, and olive oil into a blender or the cup of an immersion blender. Puree until smooth.

2. Add the pine nuts and puree again. Store in a covered container in the refrigerator for up to 3 days.

Nutrition Facts: 87 Calories | Fat 9g | Protein 1g | Carbohydrates 2g | Fiber 1g

Guacamole

Avocado is a good source of gut-healing monounsaturated fats. Unfortunately, most commercially prepared varieties contain nightshades from tomatoes and peppers. This recipe is a cinch to whip up and flavors the dip with spicy garlic and pungent ground coriander, cumin, and black peppercorns.

Yield: 8 (2-tablespoon) servings   *Prep time:* 5 minutes   *Cook time:* none

Egg-Free, Nut-Free, Allergen-Free, Vegan

1 teaspoon coriander seed	2 teaspoons minced fresh garlic
½ teaspoon peppercorns	2 tablespoons lime juice
⅛ teaspoon cumin seeds	sea salt, to taste
4 large, ripe avocados, diced	¼ cup minced fresh cilantro (optional)

1. Place the coriander, peppercorns, and cumin in a dry skillet and toast over medium heat until fragrant, about 2 minutes. Transfer to a mortar and pestle and pulverize until finely ground.

2. Add the avocado, garlic, and lime juice. Season to taste with salt. Stir in the cilantro, if using.

Nutrition Facts: 73 Calories | Fat 7g | Protein 1g | Carbohydrates 4g | Fiber 3g

Essential White Wine Vinaigrette

I haven't bought a bottle of salad dressing in... well, I can't even remember. And it's not because I'm just eager for a kitchen project. First, I like knowing the ingredients in my salad dressing and avoiding soybean oil, thickeners, and sugar. Second, it's really easy. The template is 1 part vinegar to 2 parts oil. I've included my three favorite variations here.

Yield: 8 (2-tablespoon) servings *Prep time:* 5 minutes *Cook time:* none

Egg-Free, Nut-Free, Allergen-Free, Vegan

2 tablespoons minced shallots	1 tablespoon honey
1 teaspoon minced fresh thyme	⅔ cup extra-virgin olive oil
¼ cup white wine vinegar	sea salt, to taste
2 tablespoons lemon juice	freshly ground pepper, to taste
1 teaspoon Dijon mustard	

1. Whisk the shallots, thyme, vinegar, lemon juice, mustard, and honey in a large glass measuring cup.

2. Slowly drizzle in the olive oil, whisking constantly. Season with salt and pepper.

Tip: You can also prepare this dressing in a glass jar. Add all of the ingredients, cover tightly with a lid, and shake vigorously to combine.

Nutrition Facts: 177 Calories | Fat 19g | Protein 0g | Carbohydrates 3g | Fiber 0g

Soy Ginger Asian Dressing

Avocado oil has a more neutral flavor than olive oil, so I have used that in this recipe. If olive oil is all you have, it will work just fine.

Yield: 8 (2-tablespoon) servings   *Prep time:* 5 minutes   *Cook time:* none

Egg-Free, Nut-Free, Vegan

1 teaspoon minced fresh ginger

1 teaspoon minced fresh garlic

2 tablespoons rice vinegar

2 tablespoons lime juice

2 tablespoons gluten-free soy sauce

1 tablespoon honey

1 tablespoon toasted sesame oil

½ cup avocado oil

sea salt, to taste

freshly ground pepper, to taste

1. Whisk the ginger, garlic, vinegar, lime juice, soy sauce, and honey in a large glass measuring cup.

2. Slowly drizzle in the sesame oil and avocado oil, whisking constantly. Season with salt and pepper.

Nutrition Facts: 177 Calories | Fat 19g | Protein 0g | Carbohydrates 3g | Fiber 0g

Balsamic Vinaigrette

Balsamic vinegar, maple syrup, and herbs make this salad dressing downright addicting. This dressing works as a marinade for meat, too!

Yield: 8 (2-tablespoon) servings   *Prep time:* 5 minutes   *Cook time:* none

Egg-Free, Nut-Free, Allergen-Free, Vegan

2 tablespoons minced shallots

1 tablespoon minced fresh basil

¼ cup balsamic vinegar

1 tablespoon maple syrup

⅔ cup extra-virgin olive oil

sea salt, to taste

freshly ground pepper, to taste

1. Whisk the shallots, basil, vinegar, and maple syrup in a large glass measuring cup.

2. Slowly drizzle in the olive oil, whisking constantly. Season with salt and pepper.

Nutrition Facts: 177 Calories | Fat 19g | Protein 0g | Carbohydrates 3g | Fiber 0g

Tomato-Free Marinara Sauce

Yes, it's possible to enjoy a marinara sauce without tomatoes. While it doesn't taste exactly like the real deal, it makes a fine substitution for those times when you're looking for familiar flavors. The red wine adds some of the acidity missing from the tomatoes, while basil, oregano, and rosemary infuse the sauce with Italian flavors.

Yield: 4 (½-cup) servings   *Prep time:* 5 minutes   *Cook time:* 23 minutes

Egg-Free, Nut-Free, Allergen-Free

2 tablespoons extra-virgin olive oil

1 onion, minced

3 cloves garlic, minced

1 cup diced carrots

½ cup diced beets (about 1 small beet)

½ cup diced sweet potato

¼ cup red wine (optional)

1 cup Chicken Broth (page 171)

1 teaspoons minced fresh oregano

1 teaspoon minced fresh rosemary

sea salt, to taste

freshly ground pepper, to taste

2 tablespoons minced fresh basil

1. Heat the oil in a medium pot over medium heat. Cook the onion for 5 minutes. Add the garlic and cook for another minute, until fragrant.

2. Add the carrots, beets, and sweet potato, and cook for 1 minute.

3. Add the red wine, if using, and cook for 1 minute to evaporate some of the alcohol.

4. Add the chicken broth, oregano, and rosemary. Season generously with salt and pepper. Simmer for 15 minutes, until the vegetables are tender. Use an immersion blender to puree until mostly smooth. Stir in the fresh basil.

Nutrition Facts: 112 Calories | Fat 7g | Protein 1g | Carbohydrates 10g | Fiber 2g

Almond Milk

Many of the recipes in this book call for unsweetened almond milk. I like to make it without vanilla so that I can use it in savory recipes. But, feel free to add a couple dates and a splash of vanilla extract to the blender if you know you'll be using it for baking or smoothies.

Yield: 4 cups (32 ounces)   *Prep time:* 5 minutes, plus 1 hour to soak   *Cook time:* none

Egg-Free, Vegan

1 cup raw almonds

4 cups water, divided, plus more to soak

pinch sea salt

1. Soak the almonds in water for at least 1 hour, but not more than 24 hours.

2. Add the almonds and 1 cup of water to a blender. Puree until smooth. Add the remaining water and salt and blend for 1 minute.

3. Pour the mixture through a nut-milk bag and squeeze the bag to extract all of the liquid.

4. Store in a covered container in the refrigerator for up to 5 days.

Nutrition Facts: 30 Calories | Fat 3g | Protein 1g | Carbohydrates 1g | Fiber 0g

Macadamia Nut Cheese

This fluffy nut mixture can be used as a cheese filling in savory dishes or sweetened with a bit of sugar for a sweet ricotta. See below for variations.

Yield: 8 (2-tablespoon) servings   *Prep time:* 5 minutes   *Cook time:* none
Egg-Free, Vegan

1 cup macadamia nuts

¼ to ½ cup water

1 tablespoon lemon juice

¾ teaspoon sea salt

1. Place the nuts, ¼ cup of water, lemon juice, and sea salt in a blender and puree until smooth, adding additional water as necessary.

Tip: Make the nuts easier to blend by soaking them in hot water for 1 hour. Rinse and drain before using.

Nutrition Facts: 120 Calories | Fat 13g | Protein 1g | Carbohydrates 2g | Fiber 1g

Shallot and Herb Macadamia Cheese: Use this savory cheese as a topping for grain-free crackers or as you would on a typical cheese board. Add 2 tablespoons minced shallots, 1 tablespoon minced tarragon, and 1 minced garlic clove to the recipe above. Puree until smooth. Basil, parsley, and thyme are fine substitutions for tarragon, if you prefer.

Nutrition Facts: 123 Calories | Fat 13g | Protein 1g | Carbohydrates 3g | Fiber 1g

Sweet Vanilla Macadamia Mousse: Add 1 teaspoon vanilla extract and 2 tablespoons maple syrup to the recipe above. Puree until smooth. Serve with Crepes with Strawberries and Macadamia Mousse (page 22), or simply serve atop a bowl of fresh berries for a delicious dessert.

Nutrition Facts: 134 Calories | Fat 13g | Protein 1g | Carbohydrates 6g | Fiber 1g

Chicken Broth

Homemade chicken broth forms the basis of many of my soups. I make it with bones and meat, so technically it is both a broth and a stock. Whatever you call it, it's delicious! Make up a large batch and then freeze unused portions in separate containers to use as you need it.

Yield: 12 (1-cup) servings   *Prep time:* 5 minutes   *Cook time:* 1 to 2 hours
Egg-Free, Nut-Free, Allergen-Free

> 1½ pounds chicken bones and ligaments
>
> 4 quarts water
>
> sea salt, to taste

1. Combine all of the ingredients in a large pot over medium heat. Bring to a simmer and cook for 1 to 2 hours, until the broth reaches the desired flavor. It will reduce by about 1 quart as you cook it.

2. Strain the broth and discard the cooked chicken. Store in a covered container in the refrigerator for up to 5 days.

Tip: For extra flavor, roast the bones in a 400°F oven for 30 minutes or until well browned before proceeding with the recipe.

Nutrition Facts: 13 Calories | Fat 1g | Protein 1g | Carbohydrates 0g | Fiber 0g

Vegetable Broth

Store-bought vegetable broth usually contains nightshades and rarely tastes very good. I make my own vegetable stock with leftover vegetable scraps saved in the freezer over several weeks. Whenever I'm ready to make soup, I simply toss everything into a stockpot and cook it. The version below calls for specific vegetables, but feel free to use whatever you have on hand.

Yield: 12 (1-cup) servings   *Prep time:* 5 minutes   *Cook time:* 40 minutes
Egg-Free, Nut-Free, Allergen-Free, Vegan

1 tablespoon extra-virgin olive oil

1 large onion, quartered

1 leek, halved and carefully rinsed

2 carrots, cut into 2-inch pieces

2 celery stalks, cut into 2-inch pieces

4 cloves garlic, smashed

1 small turnip, quartered

1 sprig fresh thyme

1 bay leaf

4 peppercorns

4 quarts water

1 teaspoon sea salt

1. Heat the olive oil in a large pot over medium-high heat. Brown the onion, leek, carrots, and celery until browned.

2. Add the garlic, turnip, thyme, bay leaf, peppercorns, water, and sea salt. Bring to a simmer and cook for 40 minutes, or until it reaches the desired flavor intensity. Strain the broth and discard the cooked vegetables. Store in a covered container in the refrigerator for up to 5 days.

Nutrition Facts: 5 Calories | Fat <1g | Protein 0g | Carbohydrates <1g | Fiber 0g

Gravy

Thickening gravy without flour is a delicate task. Grain-based flours and cornstarch are out. Arrowroot is one option, but the gravy cannot be reheated. Tapioca starch works, but too much can yield a gummy texture. I prefer a combination of coconut flour and tapioca starch.

Yield: 8 (¼-cup) servings   *Prep time:* 5 minutes   *Cook time:* 5 minutes

Egg-Free, Nut-Free, Allergen-Free

3 tablespoons canola or light olive oil

1 tablespoon tapioca starch

2 tablespoons coconut flour

2 cups Chicken Broth (page 171)

sea salt, to taste

freshly ground pepper, to taste

1. In a small saucepan over medium heat, heat the oil. Stir in the tapioca starch and coconut flours. Whisk until no lumps remain.

2. Cook for 2 minutes.

3. All at once, add the broth, whisking vigorously.

4. Cook until thickened, about 2 minutes. Season with salt and pepper.

Tip: If you have pan drippings from cooking a whole chicken or turkey, add those to the gravy just before adding the broth.

Nutrition Facts: 58 Calories | Fat 6g | Protein 1g | Carbohydrates 2g | Fiber 1g

Roasted Garlic

I like to use roasted garlic as a topping for pizza or to infuse cream sauces with flavor, especially my Creamy Chicken Fettuccine Alfredo (page 109). Plan to roast garlic when you're finished using the oven for something else.

Yield: 1 head (16 cloves, 1 clove per serving)   *Prep time:* 5 minutes
Cook time: 40 minutes

Egg-Free, Nut-Free, Allergen-Free, Vegan

   1 head garlic

   1 teaspoon extra-virgin olive oil

1. Preheat the oven to 350°F. Slice off the top of the head of garlic to expose the tops of each garlic clove. Place the garlic on the center of a square of aluminum foil. Drizzle the olive oil over the garlic. Fold up the aluminum foil into a loose package.

2. Roast for 40 minutes, or until the garlic is tender and golden.

3. Allow to cool completely. Squeeze each clove from its papery skin. Store in a covered container in the refrigerator for up to 5 days.

Nutrition Facts: 7 Calories | Fat <1g | Protein <1g | Carbohydrates 1g | Fiber <1g

Mulled Wine Cranberry Sauce

Most cranberry sauce is so lip-puckeringly sweet that it belongs on the dessert table. This version has a more grownup flare to it and gets its sweetness from freshly squeezed orange juice and just a bit of brown sugar. Use frozen cranberries if you wish—they actually break down more easily into a sauce than fresh berries do.

Yield: 8 (¼-cup) servings   *Prep time:* 5 minutes   *Cook time:* 15 minutes

Egg-Free, Nut-Free, Allergen-Free, Vegan

1 cup freshly squeezed orange juice

¼ cup unpacked brown sugar

½ cup red wine

⅛ teaspoon allspice

16 ounces fresh cranberries

1. Heat the orange juice, brown sugar, wine, and allspice in a medium saucepan. Stir until the sugar dissolves.

2. Add the cranberries to the pan and cook for 5 minutes, until the cranberries begin to pop open, stirring frequently.

3. Reduce the heat to low and simmer for 10 minutes, without stirring. Transfer the cranberry sauce to a heat-proof container to cool. It will continue to thicken as it cools. Cover and store in the refrigerator until ready to serve.

Nutrition Facts: 74 Calories | Fat <1g | Protein 1g | Carbohydrates 17g | Fiber 3g

Maple Spiced Pecans

These wildly addicting nuts are perfect sprinkled over salads or mashed sweet potatoes. They're also good for snacking on—just be careful, they're easy to overeat!

Yield: 16 (2-tablespoon) servings   *Prep time:* 5 minutes   *Cook time:* 20 minutes

Egg-Free, Vegan

¼ cup coconut oil, melted

¼ cup maple syrup

⅛ teaspoon ground cinnamon

¼ teaspoon freshly ground pepper

½ teaspoon sea salt

2 cups pecans

1. Preheat the oven to 350°F. Line a rimmed baking sheet with parchment paper.

2. Place the coconut oil, maple syrup, cinnamon, pepper, and salt in a bowl. Whisk to combine. Add the pecans and toss to coat. Spread them out on the baking sheet.

3. Bake for 20 minutes, stirring once or twice, until just browned. Allow to cool completely on the pan before storing in a covered container.

Nutrition Facts: 141 Calories | Fat 13g | Protein 2g | Carbohydrates 5g | Fiber 1g

Savory Mixed Nuts

Think of this as the classic bar snack without the wheat and peanuts.

Yield: 16 (2-tablespoon) servings   *Prep time:* 5 minutes   *Cook time:* 20 minutes

Egg-Free, Vegan

¼ cup extra-virgin olive oil

½ teaspoon sea salt

½ teaspoon ground cumin

½ teaspoon ground coriander

½ teaspoon freshly ground pepper

2 cups mixed nuts, such as walnuts, almonds, Brazil nuts, and cashews

1. Preheat the oven to 350°F. Line a rimmed baking sheet with parchment paper.

2. Place the oil, salt, cumin, coriander, and pepper in a bowl. Whisk to combine. Add the nuts and toss to coat. Spread them out on the baking sheet.

3. Bake for 20 minutes, stirring once or twice, until just browned. Allow to cool completely on the pan before storing in a covered container.

Nutrition Facts: 128 Calories | Fat 13g | Protein 2g | Carbohydrates 2g | Fiber 1g

Za'atar

This savory spice blend adds flavor to everything from Middle Eastern Sweet Potato Avocado Toast (page 44) to chicken, fish, and salads.

Yield: ½ cup   *Prep time:* 5 minutes   *Cook time:* none

Egg-Free, Nut-Free, Allergen-Free, Vegan

2 tablespoons minced fresh thyme leaves

¼ cup toasted sesame seeds

1½ tablespoons ground sumac

1 teaspoon coarse sea salt

Combine all of the ingredients in a small jar. Cover and store in the refrigerator for up to 2 weeks.

Nutrition Facts: 26 Calories | Fat 2g | Protein 1g | Carbohydrates 1g | Fiber 1g

Seafood Seasoning Blend

This salt-free seafood seasoning blend is designed to mimic Old Bay Seasoning without the nightshades typically present in the form or paprika and red pepper flakes. Instead, I increased the black pepper, mustard powder, and allspice to turn up the heat a bit.

Yield: 5 tablespoons   *Prep time:* 5 minutes   *Cook time:* none

Egg-Free, Nut-Free, Allergen-Free, Vegan

1 tablespoon ground bay leaves

1 tablespoon ground celery seed

1 tablespoon dried parsley

1 tablespoon freshly ground pepper

2 teaspoons dry mustard

½ teaspoon ground allspice

½ teaspoon ground ginger

Combine all of the ingredients in a small jar. Mix well. Cover and store in a spice cupboard for up to 6 months.

Nutrition Facts: 2.6 Calories | Fat <1g | Protein <1g | Carbohydrates <1g | Fiber <1g

Grain-Free Fettuccine

I remember the day I discovered Cappello's gluten-free and grain-free fettuccine. It tasted just like the pasta I made before going gluten free— tender, chewy, and twirlable in a fork. I realize this recipe is in the Basics chapter and there's nothing basic about homemade pasta. It is a delicate labor of love. But, it tastes just like Cappello's, for a fraction of the cost. Also, like the store-bought version, you can freeze this and store in an air-tight plastic bag.

Serves: 2   *Prep time:* 15 minutes   *Cook time:* 90 seconds

Vegetarian

¼ cup plus 2 tablespoons tapioca starch (50 grams), plus more for dusting

¼ cup plus 2 tablespoons almond flour (45 grams)

¼ teaspoon sea salt

¼ teaspoon xanthan gum

large egg

1. Mix the tapioca starch, almond flour, sea salt, and xanthan gum in a small mixing bowl.

2. Make a well in the center of the dry ingredients and add the egg. Use a spatula to stir it around, slowly incorporating the flours until the dough comes together into a ball. Place the dough onto a sheet of parchment paper and dust lightly with tapioca starch.

3. Divide the dough into 4 to 6 pieces and cover all but one with a towel or plastic so that they do not dry out. Flatten one of the dough pieces with your hand or a rolling pin until it is about ¼ inch thick.

4. Set the pasta maker to the first setting, #1, which is the widest. Run the dough through the machine twice. If it tears, fold it back onto itself and run it through again. If it sticks, dust lightly with tapioca starch.

5. Set the pasta maker to the next setting, #2, and run the pasta dough through it twice. Reduce the setting again to #3 and run the dough through twice. You can stop at this setting for a slightly thicker noodle, or drop the setting to #4 and run it through twice more.

6. Dust the pasta sheet with tapioca starch. This will help prevent the noodles from sticking to one another once they are cut.

7. Attach the fettuccine attachment to the pasta maker and attach the hand crank. Carefully feed the flattened dough through to cut the sheet into individual noodles.

8. Lay the pasta onto the parchment sheet and allow to rest while you repeat steps 4 through 7 with the remaining dough. Be careful not to incorporate too much tapioca starch into the dough as you process it.

9. Bring a large pot of salted water to a rolling boil. Carefully slide the noodles from the parchment paper into the boiling water and quickly stir with a pasta spoon. Set a timer for 90 seconds. Stir once or twice if the noodles are sticking to one another or to the bottom of the pot.

10. Drain in a colander and transfer the noodles to the sauce or serving dish.

Nutrition Facts: 256 Calories | Fat 13g | Protein 8g | Carbohydrates 31g | Fiber 2g

Grain-Free Flatbread

This recipe has stuck with me for all kinds of different grain-free doughs. It works for breadsticks, pizza crust, and of course, a nice rustic flatbread.

Serves: 8   *Prep time:* 10 minutes   *Cook time:* 18 minutes

Vegetarian

2 teaspoons sugar

⅓ cup very hot water

1 package (2¼ teaspoons) active dry yeast

1 cup finely ground almond flour

¾ cup tapioca flour (starch)

¼ cup arrowroot powder

¾ teaspoon sea salt

1 egg white

2 teaspoons apple cider vinegar

2 tablespoons extra-virgin olive oil, divided

1. Preheat the oven to 425°F.

2. Combine the sugar and hot water in a small bowl. Stir to dissolve the sugar. Sprinkle the yeast over the top and allow to rest.

3. In a separate mixing bowl, combine the almond flour, tapioca flour, arrowroot, and sea salt.

4. Make a well in the center of the ingredients. Add the egg white, apple cider vinegar, 1 tablespoon of the olive oil, and the yeast mixture. Stir to mix.

5. Dump the dough onto a large sheet of parchment paper. Drizzle the remaining olive oil onto the dough and onto your clean hands, and press the dough out into a thick rectangle, about ½ to 1 inch thick.

6. Allow the dough to rise in a warm place for 45 minutes.

7. Bake for 18 minutes, or until it begins to turn golden brown. Allow to rest for at least 10 minutes before serving.

Nutrition Facts: 168 Calories | Fat 11g | Protein 4g | Carbohydrates 17g | Fiber 2g

Rosemary Olive Flatbread: Fold ¼ cup halved Kalamata olives into the dough and top with 1 tablespoon minced fresh rosemary.

Nutrition Facts: 178 Calories | Fat 12g | Protein 4g | Carbohydrates 18g | Fiber 2g

Roasted Garlic and Parsley Hearth Bread: In a blender, combine the cloves from one head of Roasted Garlic (page 174) with ¼ cup extra-virgin olive oil and ½ cup minced fresh parsley. Pour this mixture over the flatbread after it has risen but before baking.

Nutrition Facts: 243 Calories | Fat 18g | Protein 4g | Carbohydrates 20g | Fiber 2g

REFERENCES

Fasano, Alessio. "Zonulin and Its Regulation of Intestinal Barrier Function: The Biological Door to Inflammation, Autoimmunity, and Cancer." *Physiological Reviews* (January 2011): 151–175. doi: 10.1152/physrev.00003.2008.

Gundry, Steven. "The Plant Paradox; The Hidden Dangers in 'Healthy' Foods that Cause Disease and Weight Gain." New York: Harper Collins, 2017.

Mu, Qinghui, Jay Kirby, et al. "Leaky Gut As a Danger Signal for Autoimmune Diseases." *Frontiers in Immunology* (May 23, 2017): 598. doi: 10.3389/fimmu.2017.00598.

Nachbar, Martin., et al. "Lectins in the U.S. Diet: Isolation and Characterization of a Lectin from the Tomato." *The Journal of Biological Chemistry* (March 1980): 2056–2061. http://www.jbc.org/content/255/5/2056.short.

Neimark, J. "Doctors Once Thought Bananas Cured Celiac Disease. They Saved Kids' Lives — At a Cost" National Public Radio, (May 24, 2017). http://www.npr.org/sections/thesalt/2017/05/24/529527564/doctors-once-thought-bananas-cured-celiac-disease-it-saved-kids-lives-at-a-cost.

Patel, Bijal, et al. "Potato Glycoalkaloids Adversely Affect Intestinal Permeability and Aggravate Inflammatory Bowel Disease." *Inflammatory Bowel Disease* (September 2002): 340–346. doi: 10.1097/00054725-200209000-00005.

Pusztai, Arpad. "Characteristics and Consequences of Interactions of Lectins with The Intestinal Mucosa." *Archivos Latinoamericanos de Nutricion* (December 1996): 10S–15S. https://www.ncbi.nlm.nih.gov/pubmed/9137632.

Vasconcelos, Ilka M., and José Tadeu A. Oliveira. "Antinutritional Properties of Plant Lectins." *Toxicon* 44, no. 4 (September 2004): 385–403. doi: 10.1016/j.toxicon.2004.05.005.

Vojdani, Aristo. "Lectins, Agglutinins, and Their Roles in Auto-immune Reactivities." *Alternative Therapies in Health and Medicine* 21 (2015): 46–51. https://www.ncbi.nlm.nih.gov/pubmed/25599185.

CONVERSIONS

Common Conversions

1 gallon = 4 quarts = 8 pints = 16 cups = 128 fluid ounces = 3.8 liters
1 quart = 2 pints = 4 cups = 32 ounces = .95 liter
1 pint = 2 cups = 16 ounces = 480 ml
1 cup = 8 ounces = 240 ml
¼ cup = 4 tablespoons = 12 teaspoons = 2 ounces = 60 ml
1 tablespoon = 3 teaspoons = ½ fluid ounce = 15 ml

Temperature Conversions

Fahrenheit (°F)	Celsius (°C)
200°F	95°C
225°F	110°C
250°F	120°C
275°F	135°C
300°F	150°C
325°F	165°C
350°F	175°C
375°F	190°C
400°F	200°C
425°F	220°C
450°F	230°C
475°F	245°C

Volume Conversions

US	US equivalent	Metric
1 tablespoon (3 teaspoons)	½ fluid ounce	15 milliliters
¼ cup	2 fluid ounces	60 milliliters
⅓ cup	3 fluid ounces	90 milliliters
½ cup	4 fluid ounces	120 milliliters
⅔ cup	5 fluid ounces	150 milliliters
¾ cup	6 fluid ounces	180 milliliters
1 cup	8 fluid ounces	240 milliliters
2 cups	16 fluid ounces	480 milliliters

Weight Conversions

US	Metric
½ ounce	15 grams
1 ounce	30 grams
2 ounces	60 grams
¼ pound	115 grams
⅓ pound	150 grams
½ pound	225 grams
¾ pound	350 grams
1 pound	450 grams

ABOUT THE AUTHOR

Pamela Ellgen is the author of more than a dozen cookbooks, including *Cast Iron Paleo*, *The Gluten-Free Cookbook for Families*, and *The Microbiome Cookbook*. Her work has been featured in *Outside Magazine*, *Huffington Post*, LIVESTRONG, the *Portland Tribune*, *Edible Publications*, and *Darling Magazine*. Pamela lives in Santa Barbara, California, with her husband and two sons. You can find her online at www.surfgirleats.com